POWER HOUSE

Elevate Your Energy, Optimize Your Health,
and Supercharge Your Performance

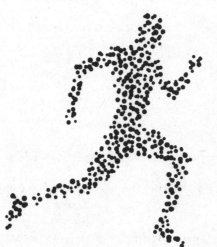

GREG WELLS, Ph.D.

Collins

Published by Collins, an imprint of HarperCollins Publishers Ltd

First edition

HarperCollins books may be purchased for educational, business,
or sales promotional use through our Special Markets Department.

HarperCollins Publishers Ltd
Bay Adelaide Centre, East Tower
22 Adelaide Street West, 41st Floor
Toronto, Ontario, Canada
M5H 4E3

www.harpercollins.ca

Library and Archives Canada Cataloguing in Publication

Title: Powerhouse : elevate your energy, optimize your health,
and supercharge your performance / Greg Wells, Ph.D.
Names: Wells, Greg, 1971- author.
Description: Includes bibliographical references and index.
Identifiers: Canadiana (print) 20220475415 | Canadiana (ebook) 20220475466 |
ISBN 9781443466714 (softcover) | ISBN 9781443466721 (EPUB)
Subjects: LCSH: Health. | LCSH: Breathing exercises. | LCSH: Dietary supplements. |
LCSH: Well-being. | LCSH: Mitochondria.
Classification: LCC RA776 .W45 2023 | DDC 613—dc23

Printed and bound in the United States
23 24 25 26 27 LBC 5 4 3 2 1

For Judith, Ingrid, and Adam

ALSO BY GREG WELLS

Rest, Refocus, Recharge
The Focus Effect (with Bruce Bowser)
The Ripple Effect
Superbodies

CONTENTS

AN UPWARD SPIRAL
OF WELLNESS

We are not made up of successively enriched packets of our own parts. We are shared, rented, occupied. At the interior of our cells, driving them, providing the energy that sends us out for the improvement of each shining day, are the mitochondria.
—DR. LEWIS THOMAS

Our health and wellbeing are four billion years in the making. Around four billion years ago, vents on the ocean floor pumped heated water out into the relatively cooler ocean. The temperature gradient from hot to cold led to the creation of chemical and electrical gradients as well. These differences in temperature, chemistry, and electrical charge were the foundation for the development of membranes that exist in every life form on planet Earth today. We humans retain these gradients in all our cells.

Three billion years ago life had evolved to the point where oxygen began to be created. Another billion years of development led to the emergence of the first single-cell life forms.

One and a half billion years ago, an event happened that would change the course of all life on Earth forever. One single-cell organism engulfed another. The engulfer was a microbe that relied on sugar for energy. The engulfee was a smaller organism that used oxygen to create energy. Once the oxygen-using organism was absorbed into the sugar-using organism, a symbiotic relationship was created, and complex life on Earth exploded.[1]

After the two entities got together, the oxygen-using organism evolved over time into organelles (smaller structures within a cell) that are now known as *mitochondria*. I know you've heard of mitochondria because you probably went to high school. They are commonly referred to as "the powerhouse of the cell," a phrase first published by Philip Siekevitz in 1957. Most adults today remember this.

The symbiotic relationship between the oxygen-loving and sugar-loving organisms gave the new cell an uncommon and powerful evolutionary advantage: it could create far more chemical energy than other bacteria or archaea that existed at the time, and it could do so under more conditions.[2] This energy advantage enabled simple creatures to evolve and grow bigger, express more genes, and develop great complexity, leading eventually to humans arriving on the scene.

Almost all our human cells (except for red blood cells), whether brain, muscle, bone, or skin, have mitochondria powering them. Nearly every other life form on the planet also has mitochondria powering its cells. As your science teacher said, mitochondria are the cellular powerhouse of all life on the planet.

Quite simply, mitochondria are the key to life on Earth. They are the key to the energy we use to fuel our lives[3] and thrive. Humans have about 100,000 trillion mitochondria, and we make about two billion mitochondria every second throughout our lives.[4]

Our mitochondria are equally implicated in our good health

and in the development of the diseases that plague us. The challenge for all of us in today's world is that our modern lifestyle and environment don't do our mitochondria any favours. Lack of exercise, nature deficits, chronic stress, pollution, industrial agriculture, and unhealthy chemicals in our environment all damage our mitochondria.

Mitochondria in Health and Disease

In addition to giving life, mitochondria are also modulators of illness and disease.[5,6] Here are some—not all—of the health conditions caused or aggravated by mitochondrial dysfunction:

- Alzheimer's disease
- Autism
- Cancer
- Cardiovascular disease
- Chronic fatigue syndrome
- Dementia
- Diabetes
- Huntington's disease
- Liver disease
- Migraines
- Parkinson's disease

Most of us have, or know someone who has, one or more of these conditions. They are shockingly common, especially as we age.[7] And they are linked to how well our mitochondria function.

Here's why. Mitochondria are called power plants or powerhouses because they provide over 90% of the ATP (adenosine triphosphate) required for cell metabolism. In simple terms, ATP is what provides energy for all the processes our cells engage in. ATP captures the energy from the food we eat and then releases it to fuel everything our brains and bodies do. We need so much of it that a healthy person at rest produces their body weight in ATP every day.[8]

When our mitochondria perform optimally, they generate all the ATP we need to support our cell health, with our brains requiring about three-quarters of that energy. This is why mitochondrial dysfunction is linked to neurodegeneration, among other issues, which basically means the deterioration of the nervous system and especially the neurons in the brain. When our mitochondria underperform—which I believe is increasingly common as modern life advances—we open ourselves up to in-the-moment issues like fatigue and to chronic ill health and disease that can afflict us for years.

Too many people are on a downward spiral of illness because they do not protect and strengthen their mitochondria, which creates health conditions requiring interventions that then lead to further damage.

It is time for humanity to create an upward spiral of wellness.

From the Primordial Past to a Reimagined Future

Since mitochondria are implicated in most illnesses that afflict us, we need to consider a new path forward.

Healthy mitochondria = a healthy, thriving you. This simple human truth can help us get past all the noise and confusion in the health and wellness field. It's a lighthouse in the information storm that will light the way toward your best life—energized, productive, creative, calm, loving, and long-lived—with an extended health span, not just lifespan.

I'm a scientist, so I could talk about the science all day. And I will write about it at times throughout this book—in ways that, I hope, will inform, inspire, and excite you. But science doesn't exist in a vacuum and neither do our lives. We must take science and use it to elevate ourselves as we respond physically, mentally, and emotionally to the powerful forces around us, ranging from troubling issues like climate change and global pandemics to the nature of our workplace culture and our family lives.

I believe we're in a moment of disruption in our historical timeline, a point of significant change when, more than ever, we need to control what direction we go in. I believe we can leverage our personal energy to create positivity in the middle of all this disruption—and use it to remake our lives, redefine normal, and reimagine our future.

Right now we're stressed, we're exhausted, and we're over-whelmed. Our burnout rate is skyrocketing. We all need more energy.

In the simplest terms, we experience stressors such as social media feeds, notifications, and the news cycle with all of its rip-ples as immediate threats that add up to constant, unrelenting stress. Physiologically, that means we feel activated all the time. We have higher levels of cortisol and adrenaline coursing through our bodies over long periods. There's nothing wrong with getting a rush of adrenaline when you narrowly avoid spinning off the road after your car hits a patch of ice. There's a lot wrong with having constantly elevated stress, which has been our reality. It wreaks havoc on our minds and bodies.

Fatigue is the most immediate way we feel that chronic stress.

We're tired, even though we haven't done much. Maybe we haven't even left the house. We feel like we need to nap. We don't have the energy to cook. Managing the kids is hard. Staying connected to our intimate partners is hard. Doing a lot of things that shouldn't be hard feels overwhelming.

Most of us are in go-go hustle mode all day. We don't always eat well, rest well, focus on our real priorities, and protect time for essential recovery and regeneration. Our lives are busy, and it's challenging to prioritize our mental and physical health.

There's growing evidence that, as a culture, we've been numbing out more than ever to cope with our daily stresses: more alcohol and drug use, more social media use, more bingeing TV shows from the comfort of the couch. According to the Kaiser Family Foundation, a non-profit that tracks health issues, pretty much every indicator of ill health has increased over the past few years: anxiety, depression, difficulty sleeping or eating, substance use, worry, and stress.[9]

But I am deeply hopeful. Using the science of optimizing our mitochondria for more energy as our foundation, we can reimagine a future where we get healthy, improve our wellbeing, and flourish as we reach our true human potential.

This is a time to do things differently. We need a way to be better, healthier, more productive, more creative, more peaceful, and more focused on our wellness and the wellbeing of others. Understanding our mitochondria can light a path forward to better mind, body, emotion, and spirit.

This is a time to reimagine the future. We can create a future that is better than the past. We can improve our health and thrive; leave behind tension and stress; and create a life of calm, focused and energized wellbeing.

That's where our mitochondria come in. They will light and energize our path forward.

Protecting and Strengthening Our Mitochondria

In tying everything back to the single, most fundamental structure that powers our health and energy, I will show you exactly what to do to improve your wellbeing and perform to your potential in whatever you care about most in your life.

We can create a flourishing environment inside our bodies by both passive and active means: by avoiding some things and doing other things.

Here are some things that damage our mitochondria: exposure to pollutants, alcohol and drug use, poor diet, poor sleep, nature deficits, and lack of physical movement.[10]

Obviously, we can't always avoid things like antibiotics and NSAIDS (non-steroidal anti-inflammatories), but we *can* do quite a lot to avoid needing them in the first place. In fact, if we engage in the actions that protect and strengthen our mitochondria, it becomes less likely that we will suffer from the conditions that then require those damaging interventions.

This whole book is about protecting and strengthening your mitochondria—like how protecting a species leads to its regrowth.[11] I'll show you how you can reset and overcome the modern malaises of fatigue, burnout, illness, stress, sadness, depression, anxiety, and unfulfilled promise.

We will explore breath to oxygenate our mitochondria (chapter 1), movement to spark the creation of new mitochondria (chapter 2), energizing tactics to supercharge the mitochondria we already have (chapter 3), and thriving to leverage the power of our mitochondria to live a beautiful life of staggering potential (chapter 4). This simple holistic framework—*breathe, move, energize, and thrive*—is designed to help you reach your true potential in mind, body, emotion, and spirit.

I will show you how to leverage and optimize your mitochondria to improve every tissue in your body, from muscle cells for physical energy to white blood cells for immune system strength, neurons in the brain for peak mental performance, and endocrine organs like the adrenal gland for calm emotional power. Taking a scientific but highly practical and active approach, as outlined chapter to chapter, will build your health as well as your energy, confidence, hope, happiness, joy, and gratitude.

A better future awaits. Onwards!

DR. GREG'S POWER-UPS

In each chapter, I'll share information, tools, tactics, and strategies to help you lead a brilliant life where you reach your personal potential. To help you along the way, I'll drop in simple but powerful tactics you can use right away to help you elevate your energy (hence the "power-*up*"!), optimize your health, and supercharge your performance.

These power-ups are focused on micro-wins and small improvements. They might not seem like much as you read them, but when you add them to your life in tiny increments, over time you will make progress, step by step, along the journey to better health and up the mountain of your potential. Small improvements each and every day will improve your life exponentially.

Be sure to add these power-ups to your days, weeks, months,

and years and practise them with your family, friends, and community.

I share these on social media @drgregwells so you can keep learning even after you've read this book!

STANDING ON THE SHOULDERS OF GIANTS

I have been so fortunate to have spent a lot of my life with incredible people who are leaders, experts, guides, scientists, adventurers, and athletes. I have learned so much from these people I consider my dear friends and partners in elevating potential and crafting a life where everyone can have peak experiences and magic moments. Throughout this book, I'll share insights from these thought and practice leaders to add depth to your learning and provide inspiration and guidance on how we can all protect our energy, optimize our health, and reach our potential.

Dr. Marc Mitchell on How to Stick to Your New Routines

Dr. Marc Mitchell is an assistant professor at Western University who specializes in behavioural change. Marc is interested in studying health incentives and behavioural economics, physical activity promotion, and how you change behaviours to get healthier. He's applied that in cardiac rehabilitation and in e-health, mobile health, and public health interventions. Here is an excerpt from my interview with him, in which we discuss setting realistic goals for change.

Success in starting and sticking to an exercise program is about helping people set very realistic goals. The notorious New Year's resolutions to exercise five times a week . . . or even to focus on weight as an outcome are so unrealistic for so many people. But these behaviours, like

20 fewer calories or 15 more minutes of standing or moving a little bit, they're very realistic. And then you can build from there.

The physical activity guidelines say 150 minutes of exercise a week, so 30 minutes five times a week. For many that's unrealistic, especially when most people are walking fewer than 5,000 steps a day. So to ask them to do 8,000 or 10,000 steps is setting them up to fail.

Instead, asking them to do 1% more or, when it comes to walking, five minutes more, is more reasonable. People can do that.

In fact, in terms of physical activity, you get the most bang for your buck when you get somebody who does absolutely nothing, moving-wise, to do just a little bit. I call it the zero to 60. When you go from zero minutes a week to 30 minutes of activity or maybe even 60 . . . then you're doing wonderful, amazing things for your health, even if those changes don't necessarily show up on the limited vocabulary of a scale.

Listen to the complete interview on my podcast at https://bit.ly/DrMarcMitchell.

BREATHE

BREATH, OXYGEN, AND THE SOURCE OF ENERGY FOR LIFE

* *

Life is not measured by the number of breaths we take,
but by the moments that take our breath away.
—Maya Angelou

When my son, Adam, came into the world, he was so little: covered in blood, eyes closed, lips quivering. I could see his ribs heaving and his belly expanding and contracting as he struggled to bring cold air into his lungs.

Suddenly, after what seemed like an eternity as I watched him gasping, his rib cage expanded and he drew a deep breath into his belly. And he cried. It was glorious. He was breathing for his life.

I was mesmerized by Adam as he drew his first breaths. I felt joy and fascination as a parent. I watched in amazement and wonder as a physiologist and scientist.

I share this moment because it highlights the fact that our breath is the key to life. We take our first breath seconds into our life and take our last breath seconds before it ends. We can live for days without water and weeks without food. If we stop breathing, we last only minutes. Nothing is more important than moving air in and out of our lungs.

Breathing moves oxygen into our lungs and blood and removes carbon dioxide from our bodies. Oxygen gets transported in our blood—bonded to the hemoglobin in our red blood cells—to the working tissues, like our muscle cells or neuron cells in our brains. Oxygen is drawn into the cells to power our mitochondria, which then create energy in the form of adenosine triphosphate, or ATP. When we stop breathing, oxygen stops moving to our mitochondria, our energy gets used up, all cellular activity stops, and we die.

Breathing fuels our mitochondria, and mitochondria power our lives.

Being able to breathe is so important that control systems in the body will take blood away from your arms and legs and redirect it to your respiratory muscles to keep you breathing when your body is getting tired. This defence mechanism is what I studied in my Ph.D. research.[1]

When we increase our physical activity, we deepen and speed up our breathing to supply our working muscles with oxygen and to get carbon dioxide out of our blood. Movement and breathing are entwined. When we breathe better, we can perform better in our activities, from physical workouts to how well we think. But the importance of breath goes beyond just athletes breathing to power their performances. Consider the following:

- Singers and actors using their breath to share music and emotions with their audiences

- A meditator directing their attention to their breath to calm and focus the mind
- A parent giving their frightened child a hug and holding them until their breathing settles
- A speaker or presenter breathing across their vocal cords to create vibrations that carry through the air to other people who hear their words and see the world in a new way

Breathing is also critical for those who push the limits of their potential. Athletes breathe deeply to power their performances. Mountain climbers breathe deeply to oxygenate as they get close to the sky. Free divers hold their breath to explore the ocean depths without scuba gear. Swimmers and rowers must breathe in time with their movements to be able to perform to their potential.

Breath makes life, health, wellbeing, and human achievement possible. Alternatively, impaired breathing can take it all away. Many diseases affect our ability to breathe, such as asthma, cystic fibrosis, chronic obstructive pulmonary disease (COPD), and sleep apnea. So can infections like pneumonia, colds, and the flu. When we don't breathe well, total health is deeply compromised.

Breath and disease work synergistically in ways that can improve or impair our health. I have focused my research career and practice as an applied physiologist on exploring the interaction between breathing and human health and performance. Whether it was working with children with cystic fibrosis with limited lung and muscle function, patients with leukemia who struggled with blood health, athletes optimizing their performance, or adventurers climbing mountains, the process of getting oxygen out of the air and into the lungs, blood, muscles, and brain has been a constant in my career. Which means the entire spectrum of human health, wellbeing, and potential has been my passion and focus.

I find it fascinating that the magical moments in our lives often depend on breath.

BREAKTHROUGH IDEA: MITOGENESIS

Adult humans have about 100,000 trillion mitochondria, and we make about two billion mitochondria every second throughout our lives.[2]

New mitochondria can be generated by existing mitochondria through mitochondrial fission. When we increase the number of mitochondria we have in our muscle cells, our brain cells, and other cells in our bodies, we can increase our production of ATP, making our brains and bodies more vital and energetic.

Professor David Hood, a mitochondrial scientist, has shown in numerous studies from his lab at York University in Toronto, Canada, that when we exercise, our body temperature increases, oxygen gets consumed, blood becomes acidic, and then the body increases the expression of genes that code for making proteins used to assemble new mitochondria. He says, "With the very first bout of exercise, you activate signals that promote biogenesis, and at the same time, you accelerate the removal of old mitochondria and dysfunctional segments."[3]

Although stress and inflammation can harm mitochondria, exercise, quality nutrition, and sleep can benefit our mitochondria and stimulate the growth of new ones.

The creation of new mitochondria is known as *mitogenesis*.

How You Oxygenate Your Mitochondria

Mitochondria exist at the centre of the challenges, activities, and pursuits that make up your life. Using the oxygen your breathing provides, they generate ATP, which is the energy currency of the body. Your mitochondria produce your body weight in ATP each day. In the process that breaks down food to create energy, your mitochondria produce water and carbon dioxide. You exhale to get the excess carbon dioxide out of your body and into the environment. This keeps you energized and healthy.

Here's how inhaling works: When you engage your diaphragm, it contracts downward, increasing the space in your chest cavity, allowing your lungs to expand and pull air in. When contracted, the intercostal muscles between your ribs lift your rib cage and help the diaphragm. Then, the exhalation muscles (such as those all-important abs) help empty your lungs. When you exhale, the diaphragm relaxes and moves upward. Inhaling and exhaling intrinsically depend on each other. Your breathing muscles make up about 15% of the muscle mass in your body.

Breathing is the key to ensuring that our mitochondria—and therefore every tissue, cell, and physiological process—function optimally, which is what gives us quality of life. Did you know we take approximately 20,000 breaths a day, totalling about 20,000 litres of air? Twenty minutes of relaxation breathing (more on that later) has been shown to increase oxygen uptake and carbon dioxide elimination by 5% to 16%.[4] When we don't breathe well, our mindset, health, and physiology all suffer, and the result can be disease or even death.

Although our breathing feels simple in any given moment, it's quite complicated and we still don't completely understand how it's controlled. When I was defending my Ph.D. thesis, my supervisor, Dr. James Duffin from the University of Toronto, and my external examiner, Dr. Jerome Dempsey from the University of Wisconsin, had a heated discussion about whether the brain or the body was more important in controlling how we breathe. This was excellent for me, as I could just watch and not be questioned for 20 minutes during my exam. But it highlights the fact that there is still much to learn and explain when it comes to breathing and our mitochondria.

It is generally agreed that our base drive to breathe arises from the medulla in the brain stem. For example, when we sleep, this base drive ensures that we breathe even when not moving or actively thinking. This is called the resting drive.

When awake, our breath-control neurons (brain cells) increase their activity, and we breathe a bit more than when asleep. This is called the wakefulness drive.

Both the resting drive and the wakefulness drive are controlled deep within our brains; these two drives keep us breathing 24 hours a day and match breathing to our sleeping or waking metabolism. You don't need to think about resting or wakefulness breathing—they happen automatically.

When you move and exercise, your breathing increases to match your energy demands, fuelling the mitochondria in your muscles so you can keep the activity going. You have felt this if you have ever run up the stairs or sprinted to catch a bus. Your muscles work intensely, you feel some lactic acid and breathlessness, and then you breathe hard for a minute or two to recover.

This increase in breathing happens because your brain sends signals to your diaphragm and the respiratory muscles between your ribs to work to increase the ventilation in your lungs. More oxygen gets delivered to your muscles and more carbon dioxide gets moved out to the surrounding environment. All of this happens to keep your metabolism as close to homeostasis as possible. Simply put, during exercise you breathe more to keep your internal environment safe.

When your muscles work hard, they produce other waste products like lactic acid and potassium, both of which are detected by nerves that send signals back to your brain to increase your breathing even more. Your breathing during exercise has all sorts of controllers that keep it matched to what your body needs to fuel your exercise and activity.[5] If you want to feel this in action, try holding your breath while you run. It's almost impossible. Your physiology (the various drives to breathe) will quickly overwhelm your psychology (your desire to hold your breath).

Your mindset also has a powerful effect on your breathing. Think about any time you have been scared and your breaths came faster. Or when anger has led to a forceful exhalation. Stress can result in hyperventilation, sometimes even to the point of dizziness or fainting. Studies have also shown that people who merely visualize exercise increase their breathing to match what they are imagining.

In addition to your non-voluntary breathing, such as swallowing, hiccupping, sneezing, and breathing while you sleep, you can also voluntarily control your breathing. Examples include singing, delivering a speech, blowing out candles on a cake, slowing your breath during meditation, and aligning your breath to movement during yoga practice or while swimming.

Like any skill, breathing is an instrument that can be trained, but we don't need any special equipment. We just need to understand that our breath can be regulated to perform any activity, whether it's working out, walking in the woods, having an important conversation, or taking time to relax.

The Challenge: Stress and Anxiety

When we are stressed, anxious, and afraid, our breathing gets shallow and fast, almost like rapid panting. This breathing pattern can spark and modulate our "fight, flight, or freeze" stress response. Although critical to our survival in dangerous situations, this response can be crippling in our modern world. Extreme stress, fighting, running away, hyperventilating, or feeling paralyzed rarely serves us.

When we're stressed and anxious, the resulting rapid, shallow breathing leads to lower oxygen levels and higher carbon dioxide in our blood. This makes it harder to get oxygen to our mitochondria so we can create energy to deal with the life challenge. Poor mitochondrial function affects our mental health.[6] The buildup in carbon dioxide is uncomfortable—we experience this as feeling out of breath—and high carbon dioxide levels in our blood can even lead to symptoms like a panic attack.[7]

Almost all of us instinctively take a deep breath to relax. Yogis use breathing to deliberately activate or calm the body and mind. Meditators use breath to bring their attention into the present moment and change their state of being. Yoga, meditating, and practising breathwork deliberately slow down breathing frequency (how fast we take breaths). We are learning more and more how we can use breathing to elicit the relaxation response and enhance our mindset and health.[8,9]

I mentioned in the introduction that we're stressed out, maxed out, and burnt out. A 2021 study in *The Lancet* proposes that depression has risen 28% and anxiety has increased by 26%.[10] In addition, the authors found that when it comes to mental health, women have been more negatively affected than men. Women reported significantly higher levels of depression and anxiety than did men.

When it comes to the toll that stress is taking, nearly half of the participants in a 2020 study say their daily behaviour has been negatively affected and report increased tension, anger, mood swings, and yelling at loved ones.[11]

As a group, members of Generation Z (born since 1997) report a significant amount of stress. This cohort has grown up with smart phones and social media, and heavy use of social media is linked to greater anxiety, depression, and sleep disruption.[12] Compared with earlier generations, Gen Z is less concerned about "classic" teen and early-20s issues like drinking and unplanned pregnancy and more concerned with mental health, feelings of isolation, online bullying, and earning high grades.[13]

A certain amount of stress is normal and can even be positive, urging us to study for tests, prepare for presentations, train for an upcoming marathon, or just arrive on time to appointments. But when stress is elevated over long periods—as it increasingly is in modern life—our risk for serious mental and physical health problems rises. We find ourselves struggling to sleep well, increasing our substance use, experiencing more physical pain, dealing with a weakened immune system, and managing elevated blood pressure and other ailments.

We are learning that mitochondria play a pivotal role in mediating our mental health, anxiety, and depression.[14] Experiments have shown that neurons involved in anxiety-related behaviours have abnormal mitochondria that produce unusually low levels of ATP, which is the energy currency of our bodies and brains.[15] It's possible that damaged or underperforming mitochondria, with their decreased energy production, may exacerbate the stress, anxiety, and depression that many of us experience.[16]

It's a vicious circle: stress leads to ill health and damaged mitochondria, which are then not able to function normally, which leads to further damage and further ill health.[17] Anything we can do to protect the mitochondrial environment helps us escape that cycle and restore our energy, calm, productivity, focus, and wellness.

STANDING ON THE SHOULDERS OF GIANTS

Dr. Gina Di Giulio on Managing Stress and Anxiety

Dr. Gina Di Giulio is a clinical psychologist and the CEO and founder of Path-Well, an organization that provides individuals and businesses access to mental health services. She is a firm believer that there is no health without mental health and that access to mental health services shouldn't be as cumbersome and confusing as it often is.

My clients who are a bit depressed or who avoid doing things because of their anxiety will say to me, "Okay, Dr. Gina, you're telling me to do this and that, but I don't feel like doing it. How can I do something if I'm just not motivated?"

I say to them, "It's the other way around." **Action precedes motivation.** I tell my clients, "Just do something. Just do a little thing." Because deliberate action will kickstart motivation, and then motivation begets more motivation.

Just do something. Just do 1% more, and then I guarantee you, the motivation will kick in. Once that motivation is rolling, it's going to be easier and easier for you to do the things that you've been avoiding doing and might even be helpful to improve your mood and confidence.

Feeling better starts with an action. But I think too many times people think that they must do something big to feel better. [But it can be] something tiny. What can you do that requires maybe 1 or even 5% more effort from what you're doing now? That's already a win.

So start small, because it's also important for you to experience some wins and some successes, and then it does get easier. Remember that feeling better starts with an action. It does not start with motivation.

Listen to the complete interview on my podcast at https://bit.ly/DrGinaDiGiulio.

Breathe to Restore Calm, Elevate Your Energy, and Get in the Zone

Feelings come and go like clouds in a windy sky. Conscious breathing is my anchor. —ZEN BUDDHIST MONK THÍCH NHẤT HẠNH

It's unnatural and even unhealthy to never experience stress. Stress can give us a positive push. It can tell us about ourselves and our surroundings. It can get us into productive situations and out of dangerous ones. We experience stress when we are challenged, and overcoming challenges can be some of the greatest moments in our lives.

I'm not really worried about acute stress, which is short-term: packing the whole family for an overseas trip, experiencing a disappointing response to a pitch at work, hosting Thanksgiving dinner. Acute stress, when followed by rest and recharging, leads to growth. The difficulty is with chronic stress, which is long-term. That's when you remain under stress for long periods of time, like in a toxic work environment or during a pandemic. That's when your mental and physical health begin to decline. Chronic stress can make you sick.

When the stressors in our lives exceed our ability to cope, we experience fatigue and burnout, among other issues. When our challenges are manageable and periods of stress are acute rather than chronic, then we can positively adapt, improve our health, and perform to our potential.

Let's circle back to our mitochondria. Under significant and prolonged periods of stress, we run ourselves down. Our sleep is disturbed. Our immune system is compromised. We are more likely to pick up a virus or other infection—and have difficulty fighting it off. We can end up with high blood pressure, which damages our blood vessels and increases our risk of heart disease and stroke. Anxiety and depression can spike.

Part of what is happening in this scenario is that our mitochondria are unable to meet our increased energy needs. That's when our health is truly compromised, and we end up in a state of deep fatigue, burnout, and illness.

There are many ways to combat stress and restore balance in our systems—which includes restoring the function and the health of our mitochondria. You may have effective strategies in your life, like exercising, talking to a trusted friend, or even talking to yourself and using phrases like "I've been here before. I know how to manage this. I can handle this moment." Calling on your personal support team, reminding yourself of the bigger picture, maintaining perspective, and setting up positive routines around food, sleep, and physical movement are always helpful.

So is developing new skills around breathing.

Changing and controlling your breathing can interrupt the stress cycle, starting with taking a few deep breaths. Deep breathing exercises have been part of yoga practices for thousands of years, but research at Harvard's Massachusetts General Hospital documents the positive impact deep breathing has on your body's ability to deal with stress.[18] Jeffery Dusek and his colleagues showed that mind–body practices that elicit a relaxation response changed the internal physiology of the participants so profoundly that it altered gene expression.

Let's take a deeper dive into the art and science of breathing better to fuel your most productive, most satisfying, and most joyful life.

Breathwork Practices

People don't think much about breathing. Of all the things we take for granted, breathing must be number one. It's our main source of life and energy. When I started focusing on my breathing, I became a stronger athlete and was better able to control my levels of effort and pain. —LAIRD HAMILTON

Breath control is a powerful strategy you can use to improve your brain–body health, wellbeing, and performance. Controlling your breathing means deliberately changing your breathing frequency (how fast you breathe, measured in breaths per minute), breath volume (how deeply you breathe, measured in litres per breath), or a combination of both (your total ventilation, measured in litres per minute). Simply put, you can breathe faster or slower, deeper or shallower. Changing your breathing changes your life.[19]

Breath control and changing your ventilation have been shown to alter the activity in your nervous system by changing the balance between your parasympathetic nervous system (the rest and recover system) and the sympathetic system (the activation and performance system). Altering your breathing changes the function of your heart and blood vessels as well as the hormones that circulate around your body. Breathwork can also affect your brain and psychological status. When you change your breathing, you can see the brain–body connection in action.

That's what researchers at Boston University have shown.[20] They completed a small study during which people with a major depressive disorder incorporated daily yoga and coherent breathing into their lives. After 12 weeks, depressive symptoms were significantly decreased. In addition, the study subjects had increased levels of gamma-aminobutyric acid, which is a brain chemical with calming and anti-anxiety effects. The most exciting part is that a behavioural intervention can help as much as antidepressants. That's important for all of us to know as we make health decisions to improve our lives.

In Eastern traditions, the act of breathing is an essential component of most meditative and yoga practices and is a powerful tool for changing the state of consciousness. In Western traditions, it is generally accepted that breath control has benefits for health and wellbeing, including improved relaxation and stress reduction. New research is bridging the gap between East and West by mapping the neural connections between the respiratory system and various structures in the brain and the body. We are developing an anatomical and physiological framework for understanding the brain–body breathwork strategy.

The list of benefits of deliberate breathwork seems to grow daily: reduced stress, relief of anxiety and depression, decreased symptoms of insomnia and post-traumatic stress disorder, increased alertness and concentration, a boosted immune system, greater creativity, and, of course, the potential to push ourselves to our physical limits with greater aerobic capacity. Overall, breathwork can improve our wellness and life performance in all endeavours.

And we can connect all these benefits to our mitochondria. Breathwork is one way to provide the healthy environment our mitochondria need to produce the ATP that provides our life-giving energy. Loading your mitochondria with oxygen is key to maximizing that energy. I urge you to run your individual experiments with various approaches to breathing to discover for yourself what improved mitochondrial health does for your cognitive, mental, emotional, and physical performance.

In this section, I'll get hyper-practical and show you how your breathing can enhance your energy, power your workouts, help you rest and relax, improve your concentration and cognition, and bring you into the present moment to be more mindful. Breathing better fuels your mitochondria and fires up all the best aspects of your life.

In the framework that follows, I have broken down the key benefits—what I call power-ups—of better breathing: calm, mindfulness, concentration, energy, flow, movement, and joy.

Let's get inspired and breathe all this in (pun intended).

Note that breathwork is not without its risks, so avoid stretching your rib cage, diaphragm, and lungs to their limits to prevent hyperventilation, which can happen with overbreathing. As with all body work and mental training, be sure to practise within your limits. Deep breathing can lead to dizziness, light-headedness, weakness, and shortness of breath. You may want to begin under the guidance of a physiotherapist, registered kinesiologist, or certified yoga instructor, whether in person or online. Also, it's best to consult your doctor before beginning breathwork. With that said, start small, stay within your limits, and give it a try.

POWER-UP #1: BREATHE FOR CALM

Take a moment with me. Place one hand on your belly. Next, inhale deeply and fill your belly with your breath. Pause. Then exhale slowly to the count of seven. Try that once more, letting the exhale be gentle and slow. Repeat this cycle a few times.

Congratulations. You just practised mindful breathing and, in the process, calmed down your nervous system. Your sympathetic system (ready to mobilize for fight/flight/freeze responses) decreased its activity, and your parasympathetic system (keeping us calm and rested) relaxed your internal organs, hormone system, and muscles.

Practised for thousands of years, this breathing for calm has been described in yoga as "pranayama." Translated from Sanskrit, *pranayama* means "vital life force," which makes sense since controlling your breathing enhances your energy levels.

Gentle, relaxing breaths with a longer exhale than inhale increase your energy and decrease the tension in your body and brain. As you now know, the benefits of a breathwork practice like this are significant, so learning this technique can have a powerful positive effect on your health and life.

Pranayama, or controlled relaxation breathing, has three elements. The first phase is to take the breath inside the body (inhale), the second is to retain the breath (pause), and the third is to let the air out of your lungs (exhale). When we bring focused attention to breathing during this process, we practise pranayama breathing, which we can use to calm down and relax anytime, anywhere.

Let me explain this a little more with the help of some excited researchers and unusually Zen mice. Many years ago, it was discovered that about 3,000 interconnected neurons in the brain stem control most aspects of breathing. This system has been called our "respiratory pacemaker" because it is linked to different types and paces of breathing. More recently, a group of scientists has been able to identify individual neurons in the respiratory pacemaker and divide them into 65 types, the idea being that each is responsible for a type of breathing: relaxed, excited, anxious, and so on.[21]

To figure out which of those 65 types of breathing-related neurons does what, scientists disabled one type in a group of mice. In that study, the mice stopped sighing (yes, mice sigh—about 40 times per hour). In a follow-up study, those scientists disabled another type of neuron. At first, there didn't seem to be any effect. The mice just kept lazing around the cage, as they do when there's not much going on. But then they were moved to an unfamiliar space, and they still . . . lazed around. That's not what mice do in new environments. Typically, they actively and nervously sniff around. But instead, they just chilled out.

It's not that they were relaxed so they didn't need to sniff. It's that in not sniffing, they remained calm. It's their—and our—breathing that sends messages to the brain. Active sniffing with lots of short, sharp breaths arouses the brain and even makes it anxious or frantic. The job of those sniffing neurons is to ramp up the brain and put it on alert. Then a feedback loop starts: more sniffing leads to more vigilance and worry, which lead to more sniffing, which increases anxiousness, and so on.

In many instances in our lives, it would serve us well to remember these relaxed mice. The implication of this study is that rapid breathing activates the neurons in our brain that put us on alert—and that slow, deep breaths do the opposite. The brain's arousal centre remains inactivated, and so we remain calm. To be more precise, we *create* calm.

Pranayama breathing—relaxation breathing—is also known as diaphragmatic breathing, abdominal breathing, and belly breathing. For our purposes, we are simply inhaling slowly to fill our lungs by expanding our rib cage and belly and then slowly exhaling. This process may feel uncomfortable or strange the first time you try it. But if you look at a baby or young child, you'll notice this is how they breathe. It is a natural breathing pattern that we lose access to as we grow up. If we can rediscover it, we will gain the power to control our nervous system and bring calm to our busy lives.

There are many forms of pranayama breathing, and you can learn these from an instructor in hatha yoga practices or through guided meditations. Here are a couple of simple pranayama breathing techniques you can try to get you started.

START HERE: THE 2:4:6 BREATHING TECHNIQUE

First, find a special place where you can sit comfortably or lie down. I love using my yoga mat in the middle of our music room at home.

Bring your attention to your body and breath. Place your hands on your belly.

Now inhale to a count of two, expanding your belly. Pause for a count of four. Then slowly exhale to a count of six. Each time you exhale, consciously relax your muscles and release tension from your brain and body.

Congratulations. You just completed the 2:4:6 breathing technique. It's easy to try and easy to remember. Ideally, I'd love you to work your way up to five minutes (five cycles), then 10 minutes (10 cycles), then maybe even 20 minutes (20 cycles). Don't worry about the time so much as staying relaxed and enjoying the process.

A LITTLE MORE ADVANCED: THE 3:6:9 BREATHING TECHNIQUE

In this practice, you simply spend a bit more time in the pause and exhale phases of the breath.

Find a special place where you can sit comfortably or lie down. Bring your attention to your body and breath. Place your hands on your belly.

Now inhale to a count of three, expanding your belly. Pause for a count of six. Then slowly exhale to a count of nine. Each time you exhale, consciously relax your muscles and release tension from your brain and body.

Once again, you want to gently build your skill and patience from a five-minute practice to 10 minutes and then 20 minutes of focused, controlled pranayama breathing.

As you begin with the 2:4:6 and 3:6:9 practices, you may find yourself losing focus, forgetting the steps, and thinking about "doing" things—like finishing up that report or getting the dog to the vet. This is natural and typical. Gently recall yourself back to the present and to your breath. You don't need to "banish" intruding thoughts that distract you. That sets you up for a battle against yourself, which is not conducive to relaxing. Instead, look at your thoughts as if they are objects in front of you (remember, they're mental events, not commands, and you can let them pass by). Think of an intrusive, distracting thought as a rabbit hopping across the lawn: observe and then watch it pass.

You can also engage your imagination while breathing. Imagine your breath entering you like a warm breeze passing over the earth. Pause that breeze in your mind or body and savour the wonder of it. Then release it, just as the wind blows away. Natural imagery can help you stay focused on your breath, on your internal experience, and keep the external world at bay.

The more you practise, the better you'll get. Your heart rate will slow, you'll stay connected to the present moment, and a sense of peace and calm will descend.

Use your breath any time you feel tension or stress. It will allow you to lead, stay open to input, and respond positively to life's challenges instead of reacting to them with unpredictable results.

POWER-UP #2: BREATHE FOR MINDFULNESS

We live in an era of unrelenting distraction. Our mobile devices are pinging and buzzing for our attention. Social media algorithms drag our focus to their endless scrolling feeds. An infinite number of cat videos are available for entertainment at any time.

The instant gratification and dopamine hits we have become addicted to bring us out of our present-moment awareness of our real lives and into the past, the future, and idealized depictions of fitness, fun, travel, and so much more that may or may not be real or staged.

We are now coming to realize that much of this digital distraction is essentially *mental pollution* that needs to be carefully managed and mitigated. The cost of distraction is high. The benefits of bringing your attention back to the present moment are profound and powerful. Training to learn how and where in your life you want to shine the light of your attention is the practice of mindfulness.[22] Your breath is where you can start when you want to build your mindfulness practice.

Although mindfulness has its origins in Buddhist practices, clinical research has shown that mindfulness and mindful breathing can help with chronic pain,[23,24] behaviour change,[25] migraines,[26] stress reduction,[27] building resilience,[28] and improving mental health.[29,30] Further, mindfulness training is now an accepted part of training in elite and professional sports.[31]

The foundation of mindful breathing practice is to simply focus your attention on your breath: the inhale, the pause, and the exhale. You can do this while sitting, standing, or lying down— just be comfortable.

Your eyes can be open or closed. If they are open, keep your gaze soft and don't focus on any one object.

As I mentioned already, when you practise mindful breathing, you may notice your mind wandering.[32] You may start thinking about other things, activities, or issues. This is totally natural. Try to notice when this happens, and gently bring your attention back to your breath. With practice, your mind will wander less, and you will be able to recall your attention more easily. The practice of being aware of your mind and controlling your attention is the foundation of what is often referred to as meditation.

Practising mindful breathing consistently can build your skill and capabilities, which will make implementing these practices easier in times of stress or anxiety.

Let's try some mindful breathing techniques.

START HERE: BELLY BREATHING

Using diaphragmatic breathing, or "belly breathing," is a very effective strategy for bringing your attention into the present moment and to your breath. It also has the wonderful benefit of activating your parasympathetic (rest and digest) nervous system, which calms your mind and body down.

To learn belly breathing, sit in a relaxed position or lie faceup with one hand on your navel.

As you inhale, expand your belly, pulling more air down into the lower part of the lungs. Your hand should rise as your belly expands. It's okay to expand your belly like a baby or like a statue of a Buddha.

As you exhale, contract your belly and push the air out so your hand falls and your belly returns to a resting position.

Doing this a few times throughout the day will bring your attention to your breath, help you release mental and physical tension, and lower stress and anxiety.

A LITTLE MORE ADVANCED: COUNT YOUR BREATHS

Bringing your attention to your breath has the physiological effect of lowering your heart rate and blood pressure.[33] From a psychological perspective, this practice can also help reduce burnout, exhaustion, and fatigue.[34] Fundamentally, it decreases the activity in the fight, flight, or freeze nervous system and increases the activation of the rest and recover nervous system.[35]

In addition to simply bringing your attention to the breath to gain these benefits, you can also use counting as an anchor for your mind. Here's how it can work.

Sit, stand, or lie down in a comfortable place where you can focus completely for a few minutes. Relax and bring your attention to your breath.

Take a few breaths, and simply notice the breaths passing by. Each breath will be slightly different.

Now count your breaths as they pass. You can count one on the inhale and two on the exhale, then three on the inhale and four on the exhale. You can choose to count to 10 and then start over at one, which helps keep the mind from wandering.

If you do notice that your mind has wandered, you can start back at one. Starting over at one can be done non-judgmentally. You simply notice that your mind has wandered, gently invite your attention back to your breath, and begin counting again.

It helps to set a timer for this exercise so you don't need to worry about counting cycles—you just practise for a set amount of time. Sessions of 3, 5, or 10 minutes work well.

You can perform this technique by counting breaths, and you can use beads on a bracelet to help you count. People of the Roman Catholic faith are familiar with rosary beads, and yoga practitioners are likely familiar with mala bead bracelets.

POWER-UP #3: BREATHE FOR CONCENTRATION

One reason meditation is so powerful is because of the focus on breath. During meditation (and practices such as yoga and tai chi), we are cued to take deep inhales and exhales, focusing on diaphragmatic (belly) breathing. As you now know, this type of breathing activates the parasympathetic (restful) nervous system. This parasympathetic activation slows down your heart rate and blood pressure and relaxes your body.

Deep breathing doesn't need to be saved for a formal meditation or yoga practice. Just taking a few deep, calming breaths can quickly decrease our stress levels. Once we are calm, we can bring our attention into the present moment and direct our concentration to the activities and tasks we want to accomplish. The ability to control our attention and concentration is a key factor that helps improve our mental health and supercharge our ability to perform to our potential in a world of distraction.

Research by Dr. Fay Geisler and her colleagues from the University of Greifswald in Germany illustrates what happened when participants did a breathing exercise for a few minutes before an achievement test, comparing deliberate breathwork to a simple relaxation exercise. They discovered that participants who did the breathing exercise reported fewer distracting thoughts during the achievement test and had less negative affect after the test.[36] The breathwork group also had higher heart rate variability measurements during and after the test, which is indicative of a more relaxed nervous system.

Breathing exercises can sharpen our concentration and enable us to direct our attention where we want it to go.[37] Michael Melnychuk, Ph.D. candidate at the Trinity College Institute of Neuroscience, has made some discoveries that highlight the link between breathing and the centres of the brain responsible for attention and concentration.[38] Melnychuk explains: "This study has shown that as you breathe in locus coeruleus activity is increasing slightly, and as you breathe out it decreases. Put simply this means that our attention is influenced by our breath and that it rises and falls with the cycle of respiration. It is possible that by focusing on and regulating your breathing you can optimise your attention level and likewise, by focusing on your attention level, your breathing becomes more synchronised."

The team at Trinity College Dublin reported numerous cognitive benefits: increased ability to focus, decreased mind wandering, more positive emotions, and decreased emotional reactivity. They also found that breathing directly affected the levels of noradrenaline, which is released when we are challenged, curious, and focused; this chemical can help the brain grow new connections between neurons. We are learning that the way we breathe affects the chemistry of our brains, enhancing our attention and improving our brain health.

When we practise observing the breath and bringing our attention back to it when our minds wander, we can build the capacity to stay focused on important aspects of our lives, whether that is taking an exam, doing a presentation, playing music, writing a story, or filling in a spreadsheet. Melnychuk's research shows that keeping our breathing regulated can keep us from producing too much noradrenaline, which happens when we are too stressed and can't focus. Our breathing practice can help us learn how to get into this healthy high-performance state and stay there.

START HERE: THE RESET BREATH

Practising relaxation at work or while studying is not just about stress relief and mental health. Dr. Masaki Fumoto and colleagues from the Department of Physiology, Toho University School of Medicine, conducted research showing that slow breathing with closed eyes helped practitioners shift from beta brainwave states (associated with stress and performance) to alpha brainwave states (associated with learning and strategic thinking).[39]

Here's a technique to help sharpen your concentration and attention at work or while studying.

Sit in your chair and place both feet on the floor. Sit up tall.

Bring your attention to your body and breath. Place your hands on your belly.

Now inhale to a count of two and lean upward as you expand your belly.

Look to the sky as you pause for a count of three. Add a little smile as you look to the sky.

Then slowly exhale and curl forward, and keep exhaling until you are out of breath. Each time you exhale, consciously relax your muscles and release tension from your brain and body.

Once you have the pattern set, close your eyes, and repeat this cycle five to 10 times.

A LITTLE MORE ADVANCED: ALTERNATE NOSTRIL BREATHING (NADI SHODHANA)

One type of breathing practice that is fantastic for bringing your attention into the present moment is alternate nostril breathing. This practice has been shown to improve oxygen metabolism and to reduce anxiety in students before public speaking tests.[40,41] I find it helpful for centring my mind and helping me be aware of my internal physiology.

Researcher Christina Zelano from Northwestern University has shown that different patterns of breathing through the nose can influence the activity of the amygdala and the hippocampus in the brain.[42] The amygdala is involved in controlling fear and stress responses, and the hippocampus helps manage memory and learning. Yoga, tai chi, qigong, mindfulness meditation, and alternate breathing between your nose and your mouth can all be helpful for reducing stress.

Alternate nostril breathing feels very strange at first. It gets easier with practice, and your brain and body respond in an amazing way. In this very simple technique, you simply inhale and exhale through one nostril at a time. Here's how it works.

Sit, stand, or lie down in a comfortable place where you can focus completely for a few minutes. Bring your right hand up to just in front of your face. Gently place your pointer and middle fingertips against your forehead, right on or above your eyebrows, and use them as an anchor.

Bring your right thumb to your right nostril. With your right nostril closed, gently close your eyes and exhale slowly and completely through your left nostril, then inhale slowly and completely through the left nostril.

Release your thumb from the right nostril, and then use your ring finger to gently close your left nostril. With your left nostril closed, exhale slowly and completely through your right nostril, then inhale slowly and completely through the right nostril.

You can pause briefly at the end of your inhale and at the end point of your exhale. Swap nostrils at the end of your inhales.

A smooth, consistent pattern is helpful for nostril breathing. You can try a 4-2-4-2 pattern: exhale for a count of four, pause for a count of two, inhale for a count of four, pause for a count of two (switch nostrils here at the end of your inhale).

Repeat the cycle five to 10 times, allowing your mind to follow the inhales and exhales. After a few minutes, bring your attention back to your body and the space around you. Practise a little smile, and then open your eyes and give yourself some props for doing your breath session.

Congratulations—you have just learned the practice of nadi shodhana, or alternate nostril breathing.

POWER-UP #4: BREATHE FOR ENERGY

In much the same way that slowing our breathing can lower activation, decrease stress, and help us regain our sense of calm, quickening our breathing—if done correctly—can have the opposite effect of increasing activation and increasing our energy.

If you are at all interested in breathwork, you have probably heard about Wim Hof. He is an interesting gentleman who has popularized cold-water immersion and breathwork.[43] I learned his technique when I was speaking at an event in Zurich and my friend Ian Lopatin (CEO of Spiritual Gangster clothing) took me for a dip in Lake Zurich in December. It was extremely cold and snowing, and when I did the breathing technique Ian taught me, I was able to stay in the icy water for 20 minutes. I now do this regularly in the lake by my home throughout the year. I live in Canada, and it is cold here for about eight months each year.

I learned from Ian, and through a specific breathwork practice called tum-mo breathing, that I can raise my body temperature and generate a huge amount of energy. According to Tibetan texts from the eighth century, *tum-mo* means "heat." Dr. Herbert Benson from the Harvard Medical School conducted research studies demonstrating that trained Tibetan monks are able to raise the temperature of their fingers and toes during meditation practice by up to 7 °C.[44] I certainly can't do that, but I can keep myself warm in icy cold water for a few minutes. I can imagine Tibetan monks using this technique to stay warm at altitude in the Himalayas. The good news is that research by Dr. Russell Newman shows that people with no meditation or breathwork experience can learn this technique.[45]

There are two key elements of tum-mo breathing that can increase our energy levels and be felt physiologically in the creation of an inner fire—an increase in temperature.[46] We experience a sensation of increased energy in our brains and bodies and heat production in our bodies. The two elements are a somatic (body and breathing) technique and a visualization. Dr. Maria Kozhevnikov of the National University of Singapore suggests that each element serves a specific purpose.[47] The somatic component causes thermogenesis (heat production), while the visualization is the neurocognitive component that aids in sustaining temperature increases for longer periods.

Let's learn how to activate your inner fire by learning to breathe for more energy.

START HERE: BELLOWS BREATH (BHASTRIKA BREATHING)

If you want to learn to breathe to increase your energy but tum-mo breathing seems a bit too involved for you, you can practise a much simpler but equally powerful technique called bellows breath, also known as the stimulating breath or, in Sanskrit, the bhastrika breath.

This is a traditional yoga breathing technique used to energize the body and brain, increase alertness and activation, and focus your mind. Here's how you can do it.

Sit comfortably with good posture and take a few deep breaths. Consciously relax your body and bring your attention to the here and now. Allow your mind to settle and quiet. Bring your attention to your breath.

Inhale and exhale through your nose, keeping your mouth closed and relaxed for a few breaths. Use your diaphragm to inhale and exhale, keeping your rib cage muscles relaxed.

Now inhale and exhale through your nose quickly (keeping your mouth closed). Aim for one to two cycles per second. Try this for five breath cycles and then return to natural, gentle breathing. Observe your mindset.

With practice, you can increase the number of cycles of bellows breath from five to 10 or more depending on how intense the practice is. As you practise, you can gradually build your blocks of breathing from 15 seconds up to longer periods of 60 seconds. Keep each block of bellows breathing to no more than 60 seconds, with two to three minutes of recovery between efforts.

Make sure to listen to your body as you do this practice. You are hyperventilating for short periods of time, so you might feel light-headed as you blow off carbon dioxide from your blood and lungs. If you experience this sensation, simply pause your practice and return to natural breathing for a few minutes until the discomfort passes. When you try again, experiment with slower bellows breathing with less intensity.

This practice is sometimes called yogic coffee. Try this breathing strategy instead of a cup of coffee the next time you need a boost.

Don't try bellows breathing if you are pregnant or have hypertension, epilepsy, seizures, or a panic disorder. If you are wondering whether bellows breathing is a good practice for you, check with your doctor.

A LITTLE MORE ADVANCED: TUM-MO BREATHING (THE BREATH OF FIRE)

As mentioned, this breathing technique matches a breathing pattern with mental visualization. The visualization often involves imagining a flame moving up and down your spine.

Sit comfortably with good posture and take a few deep breaths. Consciously relax your body and bring your attention to the here and now. Allow your mind to settle and quiet. Close your eyes.

Take a few moments to visualize a flame in the air just in front of your body. Now enclose that flame in a hollow balloon, with the ball of fire inside the balloon. Imagine bringing the fire inside your belly.

Keep this image active throughout the practice. When your mind wanders, gently bring your attention back to the fire.

Place your hands on your stomach so you can feel your breath of fire throughout your abdomen.

Keep visualizing the internal fire, breathing smoothly and slowly as you feel the heat in your belly.

Gently extend the spine as you inhale and relax as you exhale. Extend your spine tall and look slightly upward as you inhale, then relax your spine as you exhale so that your head returns to a neutral position. Allow your chest to expand and shoulders to drop back as you inhale. As you exhale, allow your chest and ribs to relax, and bring your shoulders back to a neutral position.

Now invite a deep inhalation through your nose, pause, and exhale strongly through rounded lips as though blowing out through a straw. Practise the inhale through nose and exhale through an imaginary straw for five cycles of breath, then relax and return to natural breathing.

Bring your attention back to your physical body and the environment around you. Open your eyes and enjoy the energy, heat, and mental activation.

This practice is a bit more complicated, so it is best to learn tum-mo breathing with the guidance of an instructor or via a breathwork app like Othership (www.othership.us/app). Once you have learned the basics, you can increase the number of times you perform the cycles of inner fire breath (visualized fire in the belly matched with inhales through your nostrils and out through an imaginary straw).

In Tibetan Buddhism, tum-mo breathing is matched to visualization exercises that involve concentrating on images of flames or fire and associating the image with parts of the body. For example, you can imagine the flame moving slowly and gently up and down your spine, one vertebra at a time from your tailbone up to the base of your skull and then back down. Alternately, you can imagine fire or rays of the sun in your hands and feet.

This technique increases your energy and activation, even if you don't get to the point of sweating. It's great to do in the morning, before a workout, or before an important event like a big presentation. Don't try this one before going to sleep. Also, because this technique changes your physiology, make sure to check with your doctor before starting this practice, especially if you have a chronic or serious health condition.

POWER-UP #5: BREATHE FOR FLOW

Perhaps you've heard of "being in the zone." It's a phrase often used to describe athletes operating at their peak. Or perhaps you're familiar with psychologist Mihaly Csikszentmihalyi's "flow state" concept. You'll recognize this state if you've ever found yourself completely absorbed in a task, have lost track of time, and have done incredible work. You eventually step out of it, like stepping out of a flowing river, and recognize that you've been in a kind of altered state.

Getting in the zone, accessing flow, working in the ideal performance state—different names for the same thing—is possible when tasks are neither too hard (creating agitation and stress) nor too easy (becoming rote and boring). We can lose track of ourselves and of time when our degree of activation lies between high (agitated) and low (bored) and when we find the task engaging.

For our purposes here, I'll use "flow" to describe that state where we function at an extraordinarily high level with minimal effort. We lose our sense of time and get lost in the moment. You have probably felt this when you were out for a run or bike ride and the exercise seemed so easy even though you were moving quickly. This can happen when presenting or teaching, where you and your audience are in perfect synchrony, and deep learning and powerful insights emerge into your awareness and the awareness of those you are sharing your knowledge with. Magic moments with friends and family often occur while we are in flow.

When we enter flow states while doing activities that are meaningful to us—travel, sports, music, drama, connecting, presenting—we have peak experiences. I want you to have moments of flow and peak experiences as often as possible in your life. To that end, I want to share how breathwork can help you enter flow states, get "into the zone," and have peak experiences on demand.

When the challenge of the task asks us to reach but not too far, fully engages our minds and emotions, and creates rather than saps energy, we're in flow or in the zone. We're relaxed yet alert, we feel confident and in control, and there's a sensation of effortlessness. We're doing our very best work.

So what does all this have to do with our breath? Just this: we can help ourselves get into a state of flow by controlling our breathing. You can use any of the breathing techniques I outline later in this chapter—so long as they are of the slow and deep variety.

The bottom line is that slow, deep breaths calm us and help reduce anxiety and stress. That is a positive, in and of itself. It's also a criterion for being in the zone. Those slow breaths relax and loosen us, release mental and muscle tension, and open us to the possibility of achieving at our highest possible level without effort.

Given that stress and agitation are barriers to entering the ideal performance zone, we can be deliberate about removing those barriers. Breathing is one way to do that.

Practise taking a few deep breaths and get relaxed and centred. Then bring your attention into the present moment and directed to the task at hand. Remind yourself of the meaning in your work and the positive impact it will have on the world. Then relax into the process. Flow won't happen all at once, and once you start making some progress, you'll experience the relaxed energy of your very own flow state.

Practise for a few moments each day and you will develop your ability to be present, expand focus, and stay in your flow state. If you are doing an activity that is meaningful to you while you are in flow—well, that is where the true magic of life lies.

START HERE: BREATHE TO MUSIC

Matching breathing to great music you love can be a powerful tool to elevate your mood, sharpen your concentration, and bring you into a state of flow.

Begin by taking a few deep breaths and allowing yourself to enjoy long exhales as you relax physically, mentally, and emotionally.

Then choose a song or album that you love, that makes you happy, and that you know very well (i.e., you have listened to it many times before).

Bring your attention to your breath and to the feeling of air moving in and out of your nostrils and airways as you enjoy your awesome music.

After a song or two, you can move into the activity, task, or project that is meaningful to you as you leave the music playing in the background. Relaxation plus breathing plus music is a combination you can leverage to perform to your potential and get into flow so you can have peak experiences.

A LITTLE MORE ADVANCED: BOX BREATHING

In stressful situations like public speaking, standing at the start line of a race, participating in a meeting, or having a heated conversation, staying calm, cool, and collected can make all the difference between positive and negative outcomes. In combat situations, it can be the difference between life and death.

Military personnel are often trained to use breathing to control their mindsets during operations. This is referred to as combat tactical breathing. Simply put, combat breathing involves counting to four for each step of the breathing process. Breathe in, count to four. Hold your breath, count to four. Exhale, count to four. Hold your breath, count to four. This helps keep the sympathetic (stress and perform) nervous system and parasympathetic (rest and recover) nervous system in balance.

This simple tactic can help you do what you need to do at the highest level under the most challenging conditions so you can respond to the pressure rather than simply react to the situation. Try it the next time you're feeling nervous about something you need to do, and watch your nervous system calm down and your mind settle and relax.

POWER-UP #6: BREATHE TO MOVE

We humans are capable of incredible feats of performance that push our mental, emotional, and physical capabilities to the absolute limits.

Free divers will hold their breath as they swim down to incredible depths below the surface of the ocean. Using weighted sleds, some divers can descend to 200 metres (almost 700 feet) on a single breath.

While some humans seek to go as deep as possible, others choose to climb to great heights. I've been to over 6,000 metres (20,000 feet), well short of the 8,000-metre peaks of places like Mount Everest. As you climb, the air thins, oxygen pressure decreases, and every step and breath become a challenge.

Powerlifters are yet another breed. They develop their lifting techniques to move huge amounts of mass using their muscles, bones, and highly trained nervous systems. As they move, their breathing is perfectly matched to the task, thereby increasing their strength, power, and stability during their lifts.

Marathon runners settle into a sustained rhythm of movement and breathe in time with their running pattern to get as much oxygen into their lungs, blood, and muscles as efficiently as possible to fuel their efforts.

What do all these activities have in common? Whether to ocean depths or mountain peaks, for seconds of maximum power or hours of endurance, the simple answer is that they all depend on breathing.

The process of breathing is often intricately intertwined in the activity, and the ability to breathe properly and to control the activity of breathing play a huge role in performance.

The respiratory muscles work to expand and compress your chest wall and diaphragm to move air in and out of your lungs. The resulting movement of air keeps oxygen, carbon dioxide, and lactic acid levels in your lungs, blood, and muscles stable and under control. Some athletes can ventilate more than 200 litres per minute during maximal exercise, an amazing feat given the size of most people's lungs.

Not all sports require moving large volumes of air during training and competition. Some rely on the ability to control the process of inspiration and expiration to perform accurately or on forcibly exhaling at the point of explosive activity to increase power. Tennis players need to exhale explosively when they hit the ball and then breathe slowly and deeply between points to recover.

Recent research has shown that breathing is critical for exercise performance and that, in addition to improving our performance, there are some breathing-related factors that can limit it.

For example, we can experience respiratory muscle fatigue.[48] This happens when the muscles that drive our breathing are overworked through long periods of heavy breathing. After some researchers intentionally induced respiratory muscle fatigue by having athletes engage in 150 minutes of sustained maximal ventilation while remaining seated, they found that the athletes were not able to run at a high speed for their typical amount of time. Just by breathing heavily, which did not include exercising, their performances deteriorated.

Why is this? It has also been shown that the harder your breathing muscles work, the less blood flows to the arms and the legs, which can decrease your exercise performance. Dr. Jerome Dempsey's lab at the University of Wisconsin first described this phenomenon, which became known as the muscle sympathetic nerve activation (MSNA) hypothesis. If you want to feel this in action, you can go for an easy jog or bike ride. Make sure your effort level is nice and comfortable. Then take 10 deep and fast breaths. Notice how the easy jog or bike ride feels so much harder in your legs. This effect can also be achieved in a wheelchair. It applies to both arm- and leg-based exercises.

Another challenge is that the lungs may not be capable of maintaining adequate blood oxygen levels during exercise. The impact of the blood's inability to take up sufficient oxygen is obvious: oxygen consumption will be compromised, and the mitochondria in your muscles will not be able to continue working. This phenomenon has been documented in a significant number of normal, healthy subjects and in nearly all highly trained endurance athletes.

Last, we have all experienced dyspnea. Dyspnea can be described as the feeling of breathlessness you experience during intense exercise, like when you run up a hill and feel out of breath at the top. The physiological purpose of dyspnea may be to protect and limit strain on the respiratory muscles. It's also just uncomfortable.

The key to making your physical activities seem easier to do, while at the same time improving your performance, is to train your breath just like you train other aspects of your activities. That way, you can avoid the limiting factors of breath while also expanding your ability and amplifying your energy.

Here are some tactics for using breathing to elevate your ability to move, be active, enjoy the sports you love, and supercharge your performance.

START HERE: SYNC YOUR LUNGS AND MUSCLES

Under natural breathing situations, your breathing is controlled by automatic systems deep in your brain that keep your breathing matched to your metabolism. You don't need to think about your breathing for this to happen—it's completely automated.

During physical activity like walking, we automatically adopt the most efficient and least costly pattern of natural breath.[49] However, we can deliberately optimize our breathing and make it more beneficial when we exercise by leveraging a phenomenon known as entrainment.

Entrainment is the matching of your breathing rhythm to your exercise movement patterns. Think about a rower. They must inhale as they lean forward to place the oar in the water. Then they exhale as they pull the oar through the water to propel the boat forward. Breathing must be entrained to the movement or the technique will fall apart and the exercise will seem extraordinarily difficult.

Similarly, swimmers must breathe in time with the stroke. If you breathe at the wrong time, you'll inhale some water. Tennis players will exhale forcefully in time with hitting the ball, then breathe as efficiently and relaxed as possible to recover between points. This same idea holds true for paddling, walking, running, cycling, most racquet sports, most combative sports, yoga, tai chi, and many other activities.

In entrained sports, the idea is to align your exhale with the muscle contraction or power move of the sport. In tennis, this means exhaling with the shot. In yoga, this means exhaling as you settle into the pose (e.g., exhaling into downward dog).

In walking, jogging, running, cycling, swimming, and paddling you will settle into a breathing rhythm that matches your movement. Experiment with different patterns to find the rhythm that makes the exercise feel easier and more relaxed.

This alignment, or entrainment, happens on all rhythmic repetitive activities. When we bring the breath into alignment with the movement, the effort required to breathe and to move both decrease, making the activity seem much easier.

Entrainment also makes it easier to drop from beta brainwave mode (our stress, anxiety, and tension mindset) into alpha brainwave mode (our learning, reflection, and strategic thinking mindset) and, eventually, even further into theta brainwave mode where creativity and ideation are accessible.[50] You can learn more about brainwaves, health, and performance in my book *Rest, Refocus, Recharge*. One reason why exercise is so good for our mental health is that spending more time in alpha and theta states helps us recover, regenerate, and recharge.

A LITTLE MORE ADVANCED:
BELLY BREATHING DURING EXERCISE

I've already mentioned diaphragmatic breathing, or belly breathing. I'll just add here that you can also use this technique during exercise, not just during relaxation or meditation activities.

Researchers at the Centre for Sports Medicine and Human Performance at Brunel University showed that the harder respiratory muscles must work, the harder leg muscles also have to work and the more they struggle in a race.[51] So they tested belly breathing as a way to better power performance. Most runners, for example, are chest breathers, which creates tension and unnecessary movement in the shoulders. Belly breathing keeps the shoulders relaxed and sends more oxygen to the muscles.

Experts suggest practising belly breathing while resting before trying it during exercise (see power-ups #1 and #2). Then, as you develop the skill, try filling your belly with air as you move your body. Once you get good at it, you should see a boost in your performance.

POWER-UP #7: BREATHE FOR JOY

Contemplative practices such as yoga, meditation, and tai chi have one thing in common: breathing during these exercises is attentively guided. These practices focus on slowing down respiration, long exhalations, diaphragmatic breathing, or paying attention to natural breaths. Numerous mental and physical health benefits, such as cardiopulmonary, inflammatory, physical, stress, and cognitive improvements, have been reported and may be attributed to controlling breathing in these contemplative practices.

From a scientific perspective, the proposed mechanisms by which breathing modulates this balance is through tonic (fast and forceful) and phasic (slow and gentle) stimulation of the vagus nerve.[52] The vagus nerve is the main nerve of the parasympathetic nervous system, and so breathing-induced vagal nerve stimulation may explain the physical, mental, and cognitive effects of contemplative practices.

If the science doesn't excite you as much as it excites me, then let me clarify that the specific effect I'm talking about in this section is joy. Joy is a fascinating topic. It's a general term that refers to a sense of happiness and pleasure—and who doesn't want more of that? It's also simultaneously an emotional and physiological state, much more than just "a nice feeling."

Here's a part of what the *Oxford Companion to Emotion and*

the Affective Sciences says about joy: "Phenomenologically, joy feels bright and light. Colours seem more vivid. Physical movements become more fluid. Smiles become difficult to suppress. Joy broadens people's attention and thinking. Such broadened thinking is thought to support the playful 'do anything' action tendency associated with joy. . . In this manner, repeated experiences of joy are thought to build people's resources for survival."[53]

Wow. That's a lot packed into a single human sensation. But that is how joy works: it emerges out of a complicated interplay between a person's psychology and physiology, and it has a dramatic impact on quality of life. We're not just looking for "a good time" when we look to increase joy in our lives—though there's nothing wrong with that. We're also experiencing ourselves and our world differently, opening up to learning and transformation, expanding our thinking and creativity, and improving our health.

So on that note, let me introduce you to some breathing activities that have the potential to bring more joy to your life.

START HERE: BREATH OF JOY

What better place to start than with a simple technique called breath of joy? Following this practice can release tensions and increase your natural life force, or "prana," thus both generating and opening yourself to receiving joy.

Here are the simple instructions:

1. Stand with your feet shoulder-width apart and arms at your sides.
2. Inhale to one-third of your lung capacity while you bring your arms up in front of your body to shoulder level, with palms facing each other.

3. Now inhale to two-thirds capacity and stretch your arms out to the sides, still at shoulder height.

4. Now inhale to full capacity and raise your arms over your head like you're reaching for the sky.

5. Finally, exhale through your mouth as you lean forward and "take a bow," with your arms stretched out to the sides and slightly behind you. As you finish this motion and exhalation, smile and laugh.

Repeat this sequence four more times, for five times in total. As you become more familiar and comfortable with the combination of breathing and movements, try closing your eyes through each sequence and focus your mind on the energy you feel circulating through your body.

Combining breathing with simple movements and a simple "clearing" visualization increases oxygen, decreases tension, improves mood and mental clarity, and invites more joy into your mind and body.

A LITTLE MORE ADVANCED: SKY BREATHING

SKY stands for Sudarshan Kriya yoga, and SKY breathing is a unique yogic breathing practice that makes use of a range of slow (calming) and rapid (stimulating) breaths. In a study to assess the benefits of SKY breathing, the authors conclude it can be a beneficial approach to treating stress, anxiety, PTSD, depression, and substance abuse.[54] In relieving these health threats, we have greater opportunities to experience the power of joy.

There are three main steps to do in sequence, which means you will have varying breathing rates separated by periods of normal breathing.

Here is the sequence:[55]

1. Ujjayi, or "victorious breath": This involves experiencing the conscious sensation of the breath touching the throat. This slow breath technique (two to four breaths per minute) increases airway resistance during inspiration and expiration and controls airflow so that each phase of the breath cycle can be prolonged to an exact count. The subjective experience is physical and mental calmness with alertness.
2. "Bellows breath": Air is rapidly inhaled and forcefully exhaled at a rate of 30 breaths per minute. It causes excitation followed by calmness.
3. "Om": Chant "om" three times with a very prolonged exhale.

Breathe to Live

When the breath is unsteady, all is unsteady; when the breath is still; all is still. Control the breath carefully. Inhalation gives strength and a controlled body. Retention gives steadiness of mind and longevity; exhalation purifies body and spirit. —GORAKSASATHAKAM

You have seen that the benefits of controlling your breathing are almost too numerous to count. And the best part is you can practise and improve your breathing anywhere, anytime. Sometimes, you will want to be in a relaxed state and have soft, gentle, easy, small breaths. Other times, you might take some deep, controlled breaths before starting a presentation. Or breathe in a rhythm that matches your movements during a workout.

Once you know what type of breath to use when, you can achieve so much more at a higher level of performance with more energy and much less tension and fatigue. If I need to relax, then obviously it's slow, deep breathing. And the same if I'm trying to fall asleep. If I'm trying to meditate, it's bringing my mind into the moment so I can focus on my breath. If I'm trying to get psyched up for sports, maybe I want to breathe a little bit harder to energize myself. If I want to deliver a line better when I'm speaking, I'll slow down so I can exhale as I say it. There's no one best breath. The key is using the right breath to do what you need to do at the highest level.

Whatever breathing techniques you decide to use to elevate your performance and achieve the life you deserve, I think you will be amazed by how much control you are able to exercise over achieving calm, elevating mindfulness, increasing concentration, boosting energy, getting into a flow state, supercharging your movement, and experiencing more joy.

We can breathe better to power every moment in our lives.

STANDING ON THE SHOULDERS OF GIANTS

Dr. Sarah Sarkis on Flow States

Dr. Sarah Sarkis is the senior director of psychology and performance at Exos, a licensed clinical psychologist, and a certified executive coach who draws on the science of wellness. On my podcast, we talked about how our mental state influences our health and ability to perform.

A thought isn't like a thought bubble on a cartoon or a meme. Your thought sends messages to your brain that release certain neurochemicals that then interact with your cells. It's astounding when you realize that your body metabolizes the world inside of itself and around itself, and that your thoughts—for instance, negative or positive self-talk—

play a role in the physical makeup of your brain and body. We need to stop, observe ourselves, and pay attention to our mindset, because our mindset impacts our cells and genetics. When we talk about flow, we're talking about getting into solid productivity when creativity is flowing and adjacent ideas are possible. We move out of the more rigid, calculated thinking that's very linear and into lateral and adjacent thinking. Flow lies on a continuum from micro-flow states to huge flow states like people often experience at the annual Burning Man event. There are practical skills that lead to that, and a lot of it is boundary setting: making space in your life for flow to be generated. For example, carving out 90 minutes once a day when you're really tapping into focus. You can also use your body to access flow, a little bit of breathwork, a little bit of stillness. You can do a walking meditation. You can do yoga. Create an interior state of observation and stillness. And then you set clear goals and intentions.

The big component to getting into flow, even microstates of flow, is challenge. You've got to be doing something that's pushing you. You're not doing something that's so easy that you're prone to boredom and mind wandering, but you're not doing something so crazy difficult that you've now got your midbrain involved and you're panicked.

You're in that channel, that challenge channel, where you can swim in that channel for a stretch of time. We feel better because the neuro-chemicals that get released help us feel better. We are more productive, we are more creative, we feel more connected to our self.

Listen to the complete interview on my podcast at https://bit.ly/DrSarahSarkisThrive.

MOVE

MOVEMENT, OPTIMAL HEALTH, AND
EXPONENTIAL WELLBEING

· ·

We have in our hands as close to a magic bullet
for improving human health as exists in modern medicine.
All we must do is move.
—John Medina, Ph.D.

itochondria seem to be at the centre of everything to do with
my life. In my research career, I have explored how mitochondria are damaged and how to reverse that so all children can
be healthy and active and reach their unlimited human potential.

Shortly after my return to Canada following the Tour d'Afrique
cycling expedition, I had a meeting at the Hospital for Sick Children in Toronto with Dr. Allan Coates, who was the director of
respiratory medicine. Dr. Coates was interested in implementing exercise as medicine for children with cystic fibrosis (CF). I
joined his lab to help build the exercise medicine research program, and we began studying how CF results in exercise intolerance in children.

We developed a new technique using magnetic resonance imaging (MRI) to look inside the muscles of children with CF to measure how they respond to exercise. Through the generosity of a donor named Arnold Irwin, we were able to purchase an MRI-compatible cycle ergometer so we could have the children perform exercise while in the MRI machine's magnetic field.

We started making our measurements and exploring exercise intolerance in children with lung disease, and we quickly discovered that their recovery from exercise was much slower than that of healthy children.[1] Recovery from exercise is driven by mitochondria. In partnership with Dr. Ingrid Tein, who made further measurements on the muscle tissues of children with severe CF, we discovered that the mitochondria of these children were damaged by the inflammation associated with the disease.

We subsequently moved on to perform similar research on children with a variety of conditions including obesity, Turner syndrome, leukemia, and congenital heart disease. In each disease, mitochondria were affected. Other research teams have shown that mitochondria are implicated in many other diseases, including cancer, cardiopulmonary disease, diabetes, and neurodegenerative diseases like Alzheimer's.

The key point is that regardless of where you are on the spectrum of human health and performance, mitochondria matter.[2] A lot. And the best news is that the health, wellbeing, and function of your mitochondria are within your control: exercise and physical activity can spark the creation of new mitochondria and train the mitochondria you already have to function even better.

No matter where you are right now in terms of your fitness, ability to concentrate and focus, cognitive capacity, or health, your body can adapt and improve. Amazingly, much of this adaptation can be achieved through stimulating the creation of new mitochondria via mitogenesis.

When we increase our overall physical activity and perform consistent exercise, we can spark mitoplasticity, which makes our bodies and brains more efficient and effective. Dr. Mike Murphy, program leader at the UK Medical Research Council's Mitochondrial Biology Unit at the University of Cambridge, has shown that mitochondria in muscle increase significantly after just 14 days of sustained exercise.[3] If you can stick with your new exercise program for a few weeks, you will start to notice a difference.

Ultimately, when you move consistently, you get healthier, improve your wellbeing, increase your energy, and optimize your human potential.

BREAKTHROUGH IDEA:
MITOPLASTICITY

Not only can we create new mitochondria, but we can also improve the mitochondria we already have. Mitochondria are responsible for generating more than 90% of the energy we need to survive, and they can learn and grow to be more efficient, effective, and powerful.

Research by Dr. Joachim Nielsen from the Department of Sports Science and Clinical Biomechanics at the University of Southern Denmark has shown that consistent exercise increases the number and density of the membranous folds (called cristae[4]) inside mitochondria.[5] It is along these membranes that ATP is generated, which means that more ATP production, and hence more energy, is available to us.

Movement practices such as physical activity, exercise, and training all signal our mitochondria to become stronger and more powerful.

We can think of this improvement in the power of our mitochondria as *mitoplasticity*.

How Our Mitochondria Create Energy

Humans can perform amazing feats. Sprinters run down the track with astonishing speed and control. Powerlifters make hundreds of kilograms look like a sack of potatoes. Swimmers traverse an entire lake or channel against the elements. Hurdlers gracefully clear all obstacles in their way. Some basketball players even seem to defy the laws of gravity. Before muscles can produce movements by pulling on their attachments to bones, they must first obtain a source of energy to sustain such movements.

Elite athletes across all disciplines—from Usain Bolt's 100-metre dash in 9.59 seconds to Eliud Kipchoge's 2:01:09 time at the 2022 Berlin Marathon—rely on an efficient way to generate ATP inside their muscle cells to power their movement, metabolism, and recovery. Inside each of the cells in your body can be found your mitochondria, which is where oxidative phosphorylation happens.[6] Simply put, your mitochondria break down the foods you eat to create energy that you can use to do all your activities of daily living like thinking, driving, cooking, exercising, and even sleeping. So whether you're an elite sprinter, a seasoned marathoner, or just an avid gardener, you depend on your mitochondria to move your body and accomplish all the mental tasks performed by your brain.

You probably remember that picture of a bean-shaped mitochondria in your high school science textbook. Although some mitochondria look just like that, especially those in your liver, the mitochondria in your muscles look a lot more like tubular networks that are highly interconnected.[7] They even communicate with each other by shooting electrical pulses throughout your tissues to get your mitochondria to activate to precisely match the energy demands you are placing on your muscles. The exact same thing happens in the neuron cells in your brain. The better your mitochondria are connected and fused, the better they are at providing energy in the right amounts with the right timing to help you do what you want to do at the highest level you can.

Through practice, any human can increase the number, density, and power of mitochondria in any cell in the body. When students read, study, and learn, their number and density of mitochondria in brain cells increases. Runners leverage mitoplasticity, where mitochondria become more effective at creating energy to run faster. Humans are highly adaptable, and many of our incredible adaptations—playing music, creating art, climbing mountains, teaching science, and most other human passions and pursuits—are facilitated through optimization of the mitochondria in our cells.

Unfortunately, there is a catch. Your body does not maintain structures it does not use. If you don't activate a structure in your body regularly, then your body does not consider it important for survival and will break it down and use the protein components for something else considered more critical. This is, sadly, true for mitochondria as well. If you don't use them, you lose them. After as little as 14 days of physical inactivity, your body will start to break down your mitochondria.

The takeaway message here is that you have an incredible capacity for positive adaptation and growth, but you must be consistent. Small consistent wins and 1% improvements add up over time to provide you with massive results.

The Challenge: Aging and Chronic Disease

Scientists are also discovering how mitochondria are involved in something that matters to every single human on planet Earth: how long we live. Mitochondria are very important for energy and cellular processes; mitochondrial dysfunction is a distinguishing feature of aging.

Dr. Sara Adães from the University of Porto Departamento de Biologia Experimental notes that "while many things go wrong as the human body ages, the roots of the problem are at the cellular level. And, within cells, mitochondria play a key role in aging processes."[8]

Scientists are still working on understanding why we age. There are two theories of aging: one, that aging follows a genetically programmed timeline, and two, that accumulated damage to our cells, mitochondria, and DNA leads to aging and death. We can't do much about how our genes control the aging process. But we absolutely can optimize the health of and limit the damage to our cells and our mitochondria so that we live a long, healthy, thriving life. We can accomplish this by participating in activities that stimulate mitogenesis and positive mitoplasticity.

Movement is perhaps the most powerful stimulus to build and strengthen our mitochondria.[9] Consistent physical activity sparks the creation of new mitochondria, increases the size of existing mitochondria, increases the density of mitochondrial membranes where energy production takes place, and increases the number of enzymes in our mitochondria that break down the food we eat to help create more ATP.[10] Remember that ATP is the energy of our cells.

What I find most encouraging about our developing understanding about how movement builds and strengthens our mitochondria is that we don't need to do much to get these benefits. Dr. Amanda Paluch and colleagues from the Department of Kinesiology at the University of Massachusetts, followed over 2,000 adults for 10 years and found that taking more than 7,000 steps per day was associated with 50% to 70% lower risk of mortality.[11] Although you may have heard that 10,000 steps is a good goal, current science shows we don't need to get to that threshold to reap the rewards of moving more.

It also does not appear to matter what type of activity you do. Almost any leisure-type activity helps. Data from the decades-long (25 years and counting) Copenhagen City Heart Study show that people who participated in 2.5 to 4.5 hours per week of tennis, badminton, soccer, handball, cycling, swimming, jogging, calisthenics, health club activities, weightlifting, and other sports all had the lowest risk for all-cause mortality.[12] This was after adjusting for potential confounders among subgroups of age, sex, education, smoking, alcohol intake, and body mass index. Two and a half hours per week is only about 20 minutes per day.

Unfortunately, many of us find it hard to exercise and move our bodies given we have desk jobs, spend time driving, or are studying while sitting for long hours. You may have heard that "sitting is the new smoking," and we do know that physical inactivity is an independent risk factor for health problems and chronic illnesses. A study by Dr. Ulf Ekelund from the Norwegian School of Sport Sciences that used activity monitors to track people's movement found that, on average, people sit for approximately 10 hours a day and exercise moderately, such as walking, for two to three minutes a day.[13] These participants were followed for 10 years to observe death rates. It was found that people who spent more time sitting and very little time moving had a higher risk of premature death. According to the researchers, the optimal amount of exercise needed to ensure maximum longevity and improved lifespan for those who sit a lot is 35 minutes a day. So if you spend a lot of time sitting during the day, then a bit more exercise is needed so that your physical activity can serve as an effective countermeasure to all the sitting.

STANDING ON THE SHOULDERS OF GIANTS

Kari Schneider on the Training Mindset

Kari Schneider is one of the world's top exercise and strength training coaches. She has devoted her life to high performance, strength and conditioning, research, and physiology. She has worked with elite-level athletes through the Canadian Sport Centre network, including national and Olympic athletes in swimming, rhythmic gymnastics, volleyball, triathlon, soccer, football, Paralympic tennis, aerial skiing, and many more. She is also the founder of Empower Conditioning, a training centre that brings athletes and achievers to their goals in physicality, career, and life. We had a really great conversation about health and wellbeing, exercise physiology, training, and fitness. Here is an excerpt of the conversation, in which we discuss training your brain to push past discomfort—in sport or other areas of your life.

There have been thousands of instances where I've been fortunate enough to be with humans from the ages of 13 to 75 in a realm where they are maxing out. It's usually their brain that stops them before their body does. Almost everybody will say, "I think I could have gone for another 30 seconds or another minute" . . . Or the person on the chin-up test . . . didn't try for the next one and had they tried they probably could have gotten it.

What I often will say to them is that your primal brain is simply going to keep sending you thoughts no matter what, and those thoughts are going to be almost always ones to either keep you safe, keep you comfortable, make sure you're not in pain, or find the pleasure. We tend to take them as truth instead of realizing that most of those thoughts are simply to hold us right where we are. Don't go that extra little bit of discomfort, don't try something new, don't stretch yourself a little more. Where you are is just fine. That's ultimately what that whole limbic system, that primal brain, is trying to hold you to.

But we also have an ability to recognize those are just thoughts. Our higher brain, our prefrontal cortex, can see that we're just having thoughts. We can understand that we don't have to act on those thoughts. It's just your higher brain being aware of all those thoughts that are popping up, and you can choose whether to believe them or act on them.

So when thoughts are coming up during your workouts like "I can't do this" or "This really hurts" or "I can't go any longer" . . . there's one thing you can say to yourself, and it's the line "Duly noted. I hear you, brain, I know you're trying to protect me. Let's just see what we can do. Let's just see what's possible."

Listen to the complete interview on my podcast at https://bit.ly/KariSchneider.

Move to Extend Your Lifespan and Optimize Your Health Span

The physical state of our bodies can either serve or subvert the quest to create genius. —JONATHAN FIELDS, FOUNDER OF THE GOOD LIFE PROJECT

I don't want to talk too much about the global COVID-19 pandemic, but there is one important observation of that time that I want to share with you. In general, I am an optimistic and happy person. I love looking on the bright side of life whenever I can. At the beginning of the pandemic, as we were learning about the virus and the initial lockdowns were becoming less stringent, I noticed something cool. I saw families out together: playing in the park, taking walks, riding their bikes. I saw children out with their parents. I saw people of all ages moving around and getting exercise. The cool element that made me so hopeful was that all these people were of different shapes, sizes, ages, and abilities. From toddlers to grandparents, people were benefiting from being outside and moving.

The key message here is that it doesn't matter where you are on the spectrum of age, health, or fitness. Anyone and everyone can improve their health and wellbeing across their lifespan via mitogenesis (the creation of new mitochondria) and mitoplasticity (the adaptation and enhancement of our mitochondria), both of which are associated with exercising. Robert Jacobs of the Zurich Center for Integrative Human Physiology found not only that mitochondrial content (the number of mitochondria in tissue) was elevated in people with higher fitness levels but also that people who had been exercising consistently had higher levels of beta-oxidation, maximal oxidative phosphorylation, and total electron transport system capacity than less active individuals.[14] These are characteristics of mitoplasticity, or our mitochondria becoming more efficient and effective with physical activity.

Maybe you're wondering whether these athletes and fit people were just born that way. Maybe they have good genetics and that is why they are fit. Sure, there's no question that genetics plays a role in our fitness and our health. Some people are genetically gifted with the code for better endurance, flexibility, strength, and even mindset characteristics like happiness. What genes we inherit from our parents is not in our control, and neither is the mitochondrial DNA that we inherit from our mothers. However, the expression of our genetics (commonly referred to as "epigenetics") is under our control and influence. When we are consistently physically active, the amount of messenger RNA (mRNA) related to mitochondrial structure that sparks mitogenesis and the amount of mRNA related to mitochondrial enzymes that help with mitoplasticity are both elevated.[15] You can think of your inherited DNA as the post office and mRNA as the mail carriers that deliver the messages. Although the post office might not change much, you can get more mail carriers and they can get bikes to deliver more mail faster.

It doesn't matter where you are on the spectrum of the human condition. It doesn't matter how fit you are. It doesn't matter what age you are. It doesn't matter how sick you are or what illness is challenging you. You can leverage the benefits of movement to spark the creation of new mitochondria and develop the capacity of the mitochondria you already have to generate more energy, health, and wellbeing across your lifespan.

And those changes happen quickly. In as little as 10 days of regular movement, you will generate increases in mitochondrial enzymes that break down the foods you eat to create energy.[16] When you start exercising, you might feel worse and more tired at first. But stick with it for a couple of weeks and you'll start to feel better, and the exercise will feel easier and easier. You'll start to notice that all aspects of your life get easier. Walking up steps no longer causes you to breathe harder. Everything you lift feels lighter. The workday is less tiring. Focusing in class is easier. Consistent movement basically turns you into a superhero.

To summarize the benefits of exercise for longevity and to prevent chronic disease, researchers from the University of Copenhagen provided a comprehensive review of the latest research and how to best prescribe exercise to treat 26 different diseases, including psychiatric, neurological, metabolic, cardiovascular, and pulmonary diseases, as well as musculoskeletal disorders and cancer. Based on scientific evidence, the optimal type and dose of exercise are suggested for each disease. If you're interested in the nitty gritty, look online for an article by B.K. Pedersen and B. Saltin called "Exercise as Medicine—Evidence for Prescribing Exercise as Therapy in 26 Different Chronic Diseases," which is freely available.[17]

Movement Practices

It's now been shown in many studies that once you actually start moving around—even just getting up off the couch and walking around the room—the more you will want to move, and, ultimately, the more energy you will feel. —ROBERT THAYER, PH.D., CALIFORNIA STATE UNIVERSITY

You've probably heard of two different categories of exercise: aerobic and anaerobic. The word *aerobic* means "with oxygen" and *anaerobic* means "without oxygen." Aerobic exercise relies on the oxygen you breathe to produce energy, and anaerobic exercise relies on the energy stored in your muscles as fuel. Think of the difference between running and lifting weights. You get out of breath when you run beyond your limits, whereas your muscles refuse to work more once they are tapped out from curling barbells.

Daily physical activities like walking, running, and swimming—even dancing and gardening—rely on the aerobic system. The more efficiently you get oxygen out of the air and delivered to your muscles and your mitochondria, the better and healthier your overall system. Moving your body stimulates improvement in the oxygen transport pathway, which then powers your mitochondria and, as a result, your body, brain, and everything you do.

Here are the basic steps:

1. Oxygen enters your lungs through your mouth and nose.
2. Oxygen diffuses from your lungs into your red blood cells.
3. Your heart pumps this oxygenated blood through your blood vessels to your muscles.
4. The oxygen diffuses from the blood into your muscle cells.
5. Mitochondria use oxygen to break down food to produce energy.
6. Oxygen passes from the atmosphere to the lungs and pulmonary capillaries, which are the small blood vessels inside the lungs.
7. Oxygen is then transported by blood vessels to the muscles, where it is taken up by the mitochondria.
8. The partial pressure of oxygen (PO_2) gradually decreases as it goes through this pathway.

Exercise improves every step of this process. With endurance training, you build a greater lung capacity and a stronger heart. As a result, there is an increase in red blood cells and capillaries to deliver oxygen to your muscles and an increase in the number and efficiency of mitochondria to create energy. Basically, your body is better able to deliver oxygen to your muscles *and* your muscles are better able to use this oxygen to produce energy. Good circulation is important for transporting oxygen and nutrients to every cell in your body, removing waste, and helping your immune system fight off illness. Increased blood flow also extends to the brain to improve concentration, alertness, and mental clarity.

Moving your body improves the oxygen transport pathway. A better pathway means better odds against developing chronic diseases, better energy to tackle everything you hope to achieve, and better mental and physical performance. In other words, better life.

So how exactly can you do that? That's what this section is all about. I'll show you how to use movement to elevate your energy, optimize your wellbeing, and supercharge your performance. Check out the following seven power-ups for practical tips on how to move your body to fire up your mitochondria.

POWER-UP #1: MOVE FOR CALM

If you don't do any physical activity, starting a workout routine can be overwhelming. The main thing to remember is that doing even just a little bit of physical activity will have huge benefits for your physical and mental health.

To activate calm, you just need to move in repetitive patterns over a longer distance, which we call long slow distance, or LSD (no, not *that* LSD). A meandering walk is a great example. You could walk, run, jog, swim, bike, or paddle—whatever feels good. If you work away from home or have time in your work-day to add in some movement, a slow walk over your lunch break works great.

When we do those types of rhythmic, repetitive activities, we drop into theta brain waves. That's why when we are on a long walk, we start ideating and creating. We come up with new solutions to old problems.

This explains why I love walking meetings. By moving slowly, I can activate my theta waves and maximize creativity. Try it. You will be blown away by the quality of conversation, the quality of ideas, and your ability to think in an agile manner. Walking meetings versus sitting meetings are extraordinarily powerful.

It's one of the reasons why Apple CEO Tim Cook exercises in the morning before work. He practises activating his body to ensure that his brain functions to its potential.

START HERE: JUST MOVE

Here's a great thing about physical activity and movement: even if all you're doing is transitioning back and forth from the living room sofa to the lounger on the back deck, you're probably moving your body to get out there. You get the point—right? I'm not talking about training for a marathon—though there's nothing wrong with that. I'm talking about taking the dog for a walk on a local trail, puttering in the garden, or heading out to the park to check out the kids playing baseball or soccer . . . you know, moving.

There are two benefits here that build your physical and mental wellness—and the health of your mitochondria. The first is reducing the amount of sedentary time in your days. Sedentary behaviour is associated with a whole host of unfavourable health outcomes, including metabolic, vascular, and cardiac dysfunction, as well as increased all-cause mortality and risk for numerous disorders.[18]

Low- to moderate-intensity movement is fine. Short periods of low-intensity exercise, such as walking, have been shown to increase creativity,[19] promote neural plasticity and episodic memory,[20] decrease levels of pro-inflammatory markers,[21] improve sleep quality,[22] and more. In short, low-intensity exercise has significant health benefits, even at a low volume. The key to this approach is consistency, however. So instead of sitting at your desk for lunch, go for a 10- to 20-minute walk every day. Any physical activity at all helps.

Whatever you choose to do, it's better than sitting all day. "Sitting is more dangerous than smoking, kills more people than HIV, and is more treacherous than parachuting. We are sitting ourselves to death," says James Levine, professor of medicine at the Mayo Clinic, in an interview with the *LA Times*. "The chair is out to kill us."[23] Keep these words in mind as you decide how to move your body.

Start by sprinkling in movement throughout the day. Set an alarm to go off every hour to remind yourself to stand up and stretch; go for a lunchtime walk; or do a few flights of stairs in between meetings. Decreasing inactive time is the first step to becoming more active.

A LITTLE MORE ADVANCED: GO FOR AN "AWE WALK"

A hike through a sublime mountain range often creates feelings of awe—admiration, wonder, even a sense of being a small speck in a vast universe—but an everyday walk can also become an "awe walk." During an ordinary awe walk, you would pay attention to the small wonders around you. The leaves on the trees. The daisies in a garden. A small dog rolling on the grass. An awe walk combines walking, which is already healthy and boosts our mood, with an intentional focus on the beautiful elements of our environment. Awe involves getting out of your own head to notice and admire what's around you.

What's the payoff? If you combine a walk with the deliberate cultivation of awe, you collect a series of images and experiences that elevate and inspire you. If you walk without directing your attention in this way, you are likely to focus on plans, to-do lists, upcoming obligations, and so on. In a 2020 study, awe walkers reported greater happiness, less upset, and closer emotional bonds to others when compared with those taking a regular walk.[24] Bottom line: it's good to get out of your head and connect to the beauty and wonder of the world.

For many people, walking can be the perfect choice. "Brisk" will mean something different to everyone, depending on their fitness level. So it's relatively simple to choose a stride that puts you in the moderate-intensity category—a bit out of breath but not straining or gulping for air. You should be able to pick up your pace and have a simple conversation with a friend without feeling overly winded. That's what moderate means.

Here are some tips for getting the most out of a brisk walk:

- You can walk indoors or outdoors. I always encourage getting outside in nature for the extra health benefits, but the great thing about walking is that you can pretty much do it anywhere. Just avoid crowded places like the mall around holidays. No knocking other people over on your quest for brain health.

- The only equipment you need is a good pair of walking or running shoes. Unless you have specific foot-related needs, anything comfortable will be fine.

- Keep checking in to ensure you're at a brisk pace. You should be able to talk comfortably with some breathlessness. If you can't talk, you're probably at a high intensity rather than moderate intensity. If you can deliver a speech or belt out your favourite song, then you're probably going too slow.

- If you're fit but still love the brisk walk option, find a hilly outdoor route, or use a treadmill on an incline to challenge yourself just the right amount.

- Aim to create a regular habit of at least 20 minutes per day or 30 to 40 minutes every other day.

POWER-UP #2: MOVE FOR MINDFULNESS

When we exercise, we put our bodies through stress. Once we recover (and through the help of other lifestyle habits such as good nutrition and sleep), we come back stronger, faster, and more efficient than before. Our hearts are more efficient at pumping blood to the rest of our bodies. Our lung volume increases. We're better able to deliver oxygen and nutrients to our tissues. And our muscles are bigger and stronger. Inside our cells, more mitochondria are created to help break down food to generate more energy—making everything we do more efficient.

As you now know, exercise also has the power to reduce stress and anxiety, decrease the risk of depression, and improve cognitive function, making it just as important for the mind as it is for the body.

The increased pace of life, high workload (both at work and at home), and pressure to succeed has led to a world plagued by a constant state of stress. The stress response is an evolutionary adaptation to an immediate threat. Which is fine. We need that sometimes. What we don't need is to become stuck in a state of chronic stress. This causes something called stress sensitivity, which is overreacting to non-life-threatening situations. It can even lead to worrying about events or things that could occur but haven't happened yet. This problem is exacerbated by the internet and smart phones, which keep us always plugged in, always available, and always "on." Chronic stress is very hard on our bodies and is associated with health concerns, including high blood pressure, increased risk of cardiovascular disease, sleep disturbances, and mental disorders.[25]

One of the ways we can manage this stress response is through exercise. There is a time and place for that deep-burn spinning class or climbing a mountain—or even for extreme sports. But there are other options, such as those that focus on mindfulness.

What is mindfulness? One definition is that it's "the basic human ability to be fully present, aware of where we are and what we're doing, and not overly reactive or overwhelmed by what's going on around us."[26] Another is that it's "a type of meditation in which you focus on being intensely aware of what you're sensing and feeling in the moment, without interpretation or judgment."[27] For example, instead of listening to music while going for a walk, simply being in the present moment and enjoying nature. Or even noticing the feeling of the water on your skin as you're showering or paying attention to the taste of the food you're eating.

What isn't mindfulness? Planning. Problem solving. Evaluating your performance on that work team. Worrying about something you said in today's meeting—or might say in tomorrow's. Talking to your kids about how to help more around the house. Navigating long-weekend traffic to get to the cottage. Even enjoying a movie on the sofa with your bestie.

You get it. None of those ordinary life moments are about being fully present to yourself and focusing closely on your inner and outer sensations. They require dealing with external situations.

Why move your body in ways that encourage mindfulness? To relieve stress, burnout, anxiety, pain, and depression. To achieve greater balance in your thoughts and emotions. To improve your cognitive function and sleep.

START HERE: MOVING MEDITATION AND YOGA

Moving meditation is any exercise in which you're moving your body in a repetitive pattern, such as walking, running, cycling, or paddling. Simple movements at a low, consistent intensity allow your mind to relax and de-stress. You can choose any movement that works for you, from gentle, repetitive exercise you enjoy (like on a rowing machine) to simply taking a walk. Whatever you choose, leave your headphones elsewhere to be fully present and mindful.

The idea is to get into a slow, easy, regular rhythm to the point where you don't have to think much about or assess what you're doing. You want to experience the flow of your rhythm and pull your thoughts away from "the busyness of life" to your own experience: how your body feels, how the air smells, and so on. Try to coordinate your breathing with the motion. Be attentive to the movement of your body and your bodily sensations. Let go of your "busy brain."

Yoga is another good option for moving meditation. Yoga is an ancient practice that flows through a series of movements and poses to improve strength, flexibility, and balance. Although there are many different types of practices, all types of yoga focus on bringing the attention to the breath, and yoga has been shown to be effective at relieving stress.[28]

As mentioned earlier, one of our biggest sources of stress is a kind of anticipated stress or feeling of worry of what's to come. Dr. Michael Goldstein and colleagues were interested in seeing if a yogic breathing workshop could help mitigate this anticipatory stress response.[29] Students from the University of Arizona were assigned to either a yogic breathing workshop or a wellness education workshop. The yogic breathing intervention was effective at improving self-reported measures of perceived stress, social connectedness, sleep disturbances, distress, anxiety, depression, conscientiousness, self-esteem, and life satisfaction when compared with the wellness education group. What's more, the yogic breathing group also had a lower resting heart rate prior to a stressful task, suggesting that yogic breathing can help mitigate the anticipatory stress response.

If you're just getting started, look for hatha yoga classes at a local studio or online. Hatha yoga has a slow pace and is a good choice for beginners.

A LITTLE MORE ADVANCED: TAI CHI AND QIGONG

Tai chi is a Chinese martial art that is now a popular exercise to relieve stress and improve health. It involves performing a series of flowing movements while focusing on the breath. Because of the required bodily control, it's been shown to be an effective way to improve balance in the elderly.[30] Tai chi has also been shown to improve cognitive and motor function, decrease depressive symptoms and perceived stress, and improve many health conditions, including Parkinson's disease, depression, dementia, and stroke rehabilitation.[31,32] There is even some evidence to suggest that tai chi can improve immune function, although how effective it is at preventing disease remains to be determined.[33]

Qigong is another Chinese practice that has gained popularity in Western cultures. Like tai chi, it involves slow, controlled movements while focusing on the breath and being in the present moment. Qigong has been shown to have physical and mental benefits, including improved immune function and sleep quality, decreased stress and anxiety, and desensitization to stressors.[34]

Yoga, tai chi, and qigong all focus on slowing down respiration, long exhalations, diaphragmatic breathing, and paying attention to natural breaths. One hypothesis for why these practices are so effective at calming us down is that this attentive breathing stimulates the vagus nerve, which is the main nerve of the parasympathetic nervous system (the "rest and digest" system).[35] Of possibly equal importance is that during these guided practices, we are bringing complete awareness to our movements and breath and are therefore not scrolling through social media or thinking about that email we forgot to send.

This unplugging from technology, even if only for a 30-minute class, can be a powerful antidote to the culture of distraction, addiction, and stress we're living in now.

POWER-UP #3: MOVE FOR CONCENTRATION

Do you find yourself forgetting things more and more? Or feeling fuzzy-minded when you need to be clear and sharp? You may be losing your edge if you're not moving your body.

A 2021 Harvard Health article adds to the pile of scientific literature linking exercise and cognitive function and improved memory and thinking skills.[36] According to the research team, exercise boosts your memory and thinking skills by acting on the body and on the brain. It reduces insulin resistance and inflammation while encouraging the growth of new blood vessels and neurons in the brain. It also seems to increase the size of the areas of the brain that control thinking and memory. Indirectly, exercise also improves mood and sleep and reduces stress and anxiety, all of which play a part in cognitive function.

So can we leverage this mind–body connection? HIIT (high-intensity interval training) might just be the answer.

Interval training is any exercise where you vary the pace of your workout session. That means mixing short periods of hard work with periods of rest and recovery. For example, if you're an absolute beginner to exercise, you might mix some easy-paced walking with short bursts of high-speed walking. Your muscles will start to tire, and you'll get out of breath—and then you slow back down to that easy pace to recover. Rinse and repeat. Those of you who exercise more regularly can find many ways to integrate high-intensity intervals into your routine. Note that when you are in the interval your focus is on the activity because it's challenging by its very nature. That challenge brings your attention into the present.

Interval training is one of the most efficient ways to improve your overall fitness and health. It has been shown to be as effective as other modes of exercise for improving fitness, or even more so.[37] For example, one research team looked at the effects of 12 weeks of strength training, interval training, and combined strength plus interval training compared with sedentary adults.[38] The researchers discovered that while strength training increased muscle size, interval training had the greatest effect on mitochondria and protein synthesis. The improved mitochondrial function was particularly evident in the older individuals, suggesting that interval training can help stop the cellular aging process.

One reason why interval training is so good for you is that it engages both your aerobic energy system and type I muscle fibres, which are used for endurance, and your anaerobic energy systems and type II muscle fibres, which are used for power and speed. It's been suggested that interval training increases mitogenesis in both type I and type II muscle fibres—meaning it generates new mitochondria in all types of muscle fibres.[39] Even a single bout of interval training can induce mitogenesis, as a team of researchers at McMaster University found.[40]

The benefits of interval training also extend to the mind. During exercise, your brain is flooded with brain-derived neurotrophic factor (BDNF), which stimulates the growth of new neurons and can improve mental alertness, learning, and memory. Although circulating levels of BDNF are elevated for only 30 to 60 minutes before returning to baseline, studies have shown that exercise has long-term benefits on cognitive function. One hypothesis for these benefits is that repeated bouts of BDNF exposure through regular exercise continuously stimulates the brain, leading to long-term functional and structural brain adaptations.

We can use the period immediately after exercise when BDNF levels are high to maximize long-term benefits.[41] For example, doing a cognitively demanding task following exercise could increase the delivery of BDNF to the areas of the brain that are active at that time. So if you're doing interval training, especially a team sport where you're continuously engaging your mind throughout the exercise, you're getting an extra boost of cognitive benefits. By stimulating your mind and body, you're improving your brain health, stimulating neuroplasticity, and boosting your concentration over time.

START HERE: ADD HIIT TO YOUR REGULAR ROUTINE

If you want to challenge yourself a bit more but you're new to interval training, here are some keys to help you get started:

1. This type of training is a lot harder on your body than aerobic exercise. So you don't need to do any more than two or three interval workouts per week. Make sure you give yourself 48 to 72 hours of recovery between intense workouts.

2. Start small. If you're completely new to this type of training, start by just adding a little bit of intensity into a walk, jog, or bike ride. For example, maybe on a long slow run, bump up the pace until you get to the next stop sign and then slow it down again. You can do this a few times throughout the run.

3. If your joints or other health conditions prevent you from doing anything too high impact, you could walk some stairs or speed walk up a nearby hill. Aquafit is another incredible option for anyone with joint pain.

4. This type of training can take very little time. So if you find it hard to fit exercise into your schedule, this is a good option

for you. Try going for a few quick flights of stairs in between meetings or a 20-minute circuit workout before or after work. Health and fitness improvements have been measured after exercise bouts as short as 20 seconds.[42]

A LITTLE MORE ADVANCED: TRY A TEAM SPORT

If you like team sports, there are lots where you constantly change your speed to run for the ball, skate hard to the net, or make a basket. These are all forms of interval training.

Team sports can be in the form of a formal workout, such as a spinning class, or can be something as informal as playing with your kids in the park or playing a team sport that requires you to do short bursts of activity. Find out what you like and what you think you could incorporate easily into your life.

Speaking of team sports, group-based interval training has some additional psychological benefits. Working together as a team to achieve the same goal can result in group flow, a peak psychological state.[43] A team environment also creates a sense of community, shared experience, and connectedness. A sense of belonging may be one of our most basic human needs, and some research indicates it might be even more important than other lifestyle factors, such as smoking, alcohol consumption, physical activity, and obesity, in terms of our mortality risk.[44]

I have a group of friends who train together. We have an SMS chat set up, and we simply post when we have done a workout. Sometimes we post a screenshot of the data from our wearables, or the map, a cool photo, or even a short video. We have all found it helpful to see what we're all up to, and it inspires us to get out there.

Here's an interesting idea: if you engage in sports that activate you, you can also activate a sense of calm. For some people, adding stress into their activities can relieve stress overall, for a net positive effect.

"When you have a high level of emotion and then you have that release, it can have that cathartic-like experience and you kind of feel that release of tension," says Lauren M. Bylsma, an emotions expert at the University of Pittsburgh.[45]

But how can engaging feelings of fear through extreme physical activity create a sense of calm? This is what happens: Fear and aggression trigger the sympathetic nervous system, also called the flight or fight response. That's when your cortisol, blood pressure, and heart rate go up and you might also break into a sweat. In turn, that sympathetic response triggers the parasympathetic nervous system. That's the "rest and digest" system characterized by low blood pressure and heart rate, increased metabolism, and a flushing away of the stress hormone cortisol.[46]

That's a powerful one-two punch: have fun with friends, and the one-two biological process of fear relief is what leads to a sense of calm and peace.

POWER-UP #4: MOVE FOR ENERGY (RESISTANCE AND STRENGTH TRAINING)

Strength training, or resistance training, is any form of exercise in which your muscles are working against a resistance to produce force. That's a bit of a fancy way of saying moving weight around or trying to move things that don't want to move on their own—which may include your own body.

Strength training leads to musculoskeletal fitness, which is made up of three parts: muscular strength, endurance, and flexibility. And, just like cardiorespiratory endurance and flexibility, musculoskeletal fitness is an important part of overall health. Simply put, strength training can increase muscle mass and strength and improve body composition and bone health, all of which make your activities easier and more efficient. Strength training has also been shown to improve factors related to cancer, metabolic diseases, cardiovascular diseases, and dementia and is associated with a 21% lower all-cause mortality.[47,48]

Since mitochondria are responsible for aerobic energy production, many people think that aerobic exercise like running or cycling is required to improve mitochondrial function. However, studies have shown that resistance training is also effective at improving both mitochondrial quantity and quality.

One team of researchers studied the effects of 12 weeks of resistance training on young healthy men.[49] They found that, in addition to increased fat-free mass, decreased fat mass, and increased muscle strength, there was also an increase in mitochondrial respiration. Another study found that 10 weeks of strength training was just as effective at improving skeletal muscle oxidative capacity—which is the measure of a muscle's maximal capacity to use oxygen—as endurance training, making it a time-efficient mode of exercise to improve mitochondrial function, strength, balance, and quality of life.[50]

Improved mitochondrial function via resistance exercise might also help prevent the loss of muscle mass that accompanies aging.[51] Since mitochondrial dysfunction is implicated in nearly every age-related disease, and loss of muscle mass contributes to reduced strength, balance, independence, and quality of life in the elderly, strength training is an ideal form of exercise for this population.

Finally, mTOR is a protein produced during strength sessions that stimulates the production of new muscle. mTOR also acts on distant tissue such as fat, the liver, and the brain to make you healthier and may be central to improving both longevity and quality of life.[52] mTOR has also been shown to stimulate mitogenesis—the creation of new mitochondria—and boost oxidative metabolism, which is basically your ability to use oxygen to create energy.[53]

START HERE: SIMPLE STRENGTH TRAINING ACTIVITIES YOU CAN DO RIGHT AWAY

So how do you start a strength training program? A common misconception is that strength training means doing bench presses and squats at the gym. That's one option, for sure, but there are many others. Basically, strength training can be anything in which you're working against a resistance. Also, you can do pure strength workouts or combine them with endurance or high-intensity workouts for some added metabolic benefits. Choose an activity that works best for you.

You don't always need a special time, place, or even set of equipment to engage in resistance training. You can choose any location that fits the bill—including your home or neighbourhood—and even use your own body as your set of weights. Or you can get creative—for example, using soup cans as dumbbells or adding heavy books to a backpack for lower-body exercises. Yoga, gardening, and housework also all count.

There are so many variations of resistance training (also known as power training or "weights"), so you can choose a variation that works best for you.

Here are some great starter strength-building activities:

Housework. Believe it or not, even housework can count toward strength training, depending on the task. Vacuuming, laundry, and scrubbing surfaces can all give your muscles a good burn.

Hiking. Any walk in which you're gaining elevation or adjusting to varying ground can count toward strength training, as you're producing significantly greater force than with a walk on flat ground. Going uphill, you are doing mostly concentric muscle contractions (shortening your muscles), and on the way down, you're doing mostly eccentric muscle contractions (lengthening your muscles). Both are great for improving strength and health. Stairs work in the same way. Taking a break at home or the office by climbing up and down the stairs is a super simple and effective option.

Body-weight workouts. Here's another no-special-equipment option. Whether or not you have access to a gym, there are many exercises that can be done using only your body weight. You can also easily sprinkle in some body-weight exercises throughout the day. For example, do 10 push-ups a few times per day—or standing push-ups against a wall if you're just starting out. Or every time you get up from your desk, do 10 or 20 body-weight squats. Whatever works for you with the equipment (your own self), space, and time that you have.

Weights. The most classic type of strength training can also be done at home or at a gym using simple weights like dumbbells or machines. You can even use canned goods or jugs of liquids you might have in your pantry or laundry room. For a work-out, you can do anything from low weight and high repetitions to increase endurance to heavy weight and low repetitions to increase muscle mass (and everywhere in between). Especially when using weights, it's a good idea to get advice from a certified personal trainer or registered kinesiologist before performing an exercise you've never done before.

A LITTLE MORE ADVANCED: SPECIFIC ROUTINES OR ENVIRONMENTS

If you want to challenge yourself more or take up a class or a new hobby as part of your workout routine, then you open the door to a lot of other options. Tap into your current interests, or consider the people you know who enjoy some activities you would like to try. Whether you are a newbie or an expert, a first-timer or a seasoned veteran, you can reap the benefits of a fun activity—on your own or with a friend or group. Here are some options:

Circuit workouts. You can combine strength and aerobic training into a circuit workout that will keep your heart rate high the whole time. To do this, pick as many exercises as you want and then perform them in sequence with minimal rest. You can keep the weights light (or use no weight) so that your heart rate stays constantly elevated. For example, you could do (1) push-ups, (2) squats, (3) lunges, (4) back extensions, (5) lat pull-downs, (6) rowing, (7) abdominal crunches, and (8) step-ups. Do each exercise for 45 seconds and then take 15 seconds to change stations. Work your way around the circuit one to three times to create your circuit training session.

Pilates. Pilates is a guided workout that combines strength, balance, and flexibility. Its focus is on the core muscles to improve posture, alleviate pain, and prevent injuries. Find a nearby studio or online class to guide you through a practice.

Climbing. It takes an enormous amount of upper- and lower-body strength to pull yourself up a rock or ice wall. Climbing also requires balance, flexibility, and mental strength—and it's fun at the same time. Like all these activities, you could try this solo at a gym (with instruction and supervision) or join a group that climbs indoors or outdoors. Again, if you're new to this activity, be sure to take lessons first and use the right equipment.

Skiing and snowboarding. These fun winter activities can provide another sneaky strength workout. Skiing and snowboarding require a lot of strength and stability to control your body as you move down the hill.

Swimming. Although swimming is predominantly an aerobic activity, it also strengthens your muscles because you are exerting force against the water each time you take a stroke.

Paddling. Like swimming, workouts such as canoeing, kayaking, rowing, and stand-up paddleboarding require that you exert force against the water each time you take a stroke.

Obviously, you can combine some different activities to keep yourself interested or challenged, such as alternating between a summer and winter sport or just mixing it up, like taking a Pilates class once a week and mixing in some weight training or circuit training.

Whatever you decide, make choices that you enjoy. If you're having fun, you're more likely to make time for your activity and develop a healthy routine.

POWER-UP #5: MOVE FOR FLOW

Flow was first identified by Mihaly Csikszentmihalyi, who described it as a highly focused state conducive to peak performance and productivity.[54] During flow, people are so immersed in an activity that the world seems to fade away and they feel a sense of timelessness, total body awareness, and ease.[55] I'm guessing you can identify with flow moments, whether it's being completely absorbed in a task, having a spark of creativity, or just being immersed in a really engaging conversation. Unfortunately, these moments are rare and seem random. But this flow state is something you can learn to control.

According to Csikszentmihalyi, there are nine dimensions of flow:

1. Concentration on the task at hand
2. Clarity of goals
3. Transformation of time (either speeding up or slowing down)
4. Intrinsic reward (an internal, not external, reward in and of itself)
5. Direct and immediate feedback
6. Challenge–skills balance (appropriate level of challenge that can be overcome with skill)
7. Merging of actions and awareness (actions feel automatic)
8. Sense of control
9. Loss of self-consciousness (decreased self-awareness)

Researchers have developed the Flow State Scale, which uses the nine dimensions to score the intensity of flow, suggesting that flow exists on a continuum rather than as a discrete state.[56]

Additionally, of the nine dimensions of flow first described by Csikszentmihalyi, three have been identified as prerequisites of flow: clarity of goals, direct and immediate feedback (regarding progress toward goals), and challenge–skills balance. These are all directly within our control, which means we can help ourselves to activate a state of flow. And of all these prerequisites, Csikszentmihalyi identified the challenge–skills balance as the golden rule of flow. To achieve a flow state, you need to choose a task or activity that is challenging but that is not beyond your skill level. Choosing a task that is too easy results in boredom, whereas choosing an activity way beyond your skill level results in anxiety. To enter a flow state, you need to find that sweet spot somewhere between boredom and stress—when you are excited, engaged, happy, and able to perform at your best.

One of the most powerful ways to access flow is through movement. Elite athletes often describe flow states as time slowing down, or a time in which they could no longer hear the crowd, or when the performance felt easy. But you don't need to be a professional athlete to experience flow. Everyone can use movement to spark flow. And the more you practise getting into flow, the easier it will be to enter a flow state in other areas of life.

START HERE: SET THE STAGE FOR FLOW

Often, we think of flow or "getting in the zone" as a random event that happened by chance. However, you can get into flow deliberately by optimizing your mind–body connection. Here are a few ways to ease your way into a flow state more often.

Choose the right activity. When trying to get into flow, choose an activity that is challenging but not overwhelming. This isn't the time to try out a new sport or activity, but it could be the time to progress your skills. Keep in mind that once your skills improve, you might need to increase the challenge so you're maintaining the challenge–skills balance.

Do what you love. In addition to finding the right challenge, it's important to choose an activity you love, as flow is more likely to occur during intrinsically rewarding activities. You're also more likely to continue that activity if you experience flow because it's *become* intrinsically motivating. Female health care workers who experienced flow during a 12-week football (soccer) or Zumba intervention had greater adherence to physical activity 18 weeks later.[57] Experiencing flow during intrinsically rewarding activities opens you up to peak experience.

Be wary of the fear of failure. One thing that gets in the way of achieving peak moments is fear of failure. The fear that we will fail at something, and the perceived shame associated with it, prevents us from putting our best effort toward something—or potentially not even trying at all. People who fear failure are less likely to achieve a flow state, whereas people with the hope of success are more likely to achieve flow.[58]

Create your optimal environment for flow. You can learn to optimize your external and internal environment to get into a flow state more often. When running, is there certain music that allows you to get into a smooth rhythm? Maybe you need a certain environment that helps you get into flow? For example, one study found that rock climbers were able to achieve a state of flow more easily during outdoor sessions (in nature) compared with indoors.[59] Learning what type of environment you need in order to enter flow will help you create your flow state.

A LITTLE MORE ADVANCED: MASTER THE MIND–BODY CONNECTION

Now that you have a few foundational practices for increasing your ability to enter into flow more consistently, you can begin to explore how to improve your performance while in the zone.

Concentrate on the task at hand. Once you've controlled your external environment, you can practise controlling your internal environment by learning how to concentrate entirely on the task at hand and block out distractions. This will take a little bit more time. However, if you get distracted, simply acknowledge that you are getting distracted and then try to return to your focused state. Maybe you need to make some adjustments, such as moving your body or breathing deeply, to get back into flow. Simply, the more you practise controlling your attention, the better you'll be able to control your attention.

Distract yourself. How's this for a counterintuitive idea: several studies have shown that our performance improves when we think less about what we're doing.

When it comes to running, for example, focusing on external sights and sounds rather than what your body is doing makes the exercise feel easier and improves performance. Even watching a basketball game while running on a treadmill has a similar outcome.

This is still setting yourself up for being in a flow state—you are just deliberately moving your attention from an internal focus to an external focus. So try shifting your focus to something outside yourself—music, your surroundings, the sound of your breath—to improve your performance.

Practise. Getting into flow takes practice, but the more often you do it, the easier it will be. If you choose a challenging, enjoyable activity and create the right environment, you will learn to enter flow more easily, not only during exercise but in all areas of life. Flow is when we are energized, motivated, focused, happy, and able to perform at our best. Being in a flow state is powerful for your mental health and your mental performance. Learning how to enter flow using movement will help you achieve this state more often in other pursuits. It can lead to being more creative, accomplishing more with less effort, building a sense of control, and becoming happier and healthier.

POWER-UP #6: MOVE IN NATURE (SHINRIN-YOKU)

This isn't the first time I've mentioned getting outdoors—and it won't be the last. The more you understand about how and why being in a natural environment builds your health and wellness, the more likely you are to make time for Mother Nature. Plus, many of us hardly get "out there" at all. In fact, most people spend on average 90% of the day indoors, while a growing body of research suggests that physical activity performed outdoors actually has physical and mental health benefits beyond those of indoor exercise.[60]

Getting outside into natural surroundings is not only enjoyable but also good for your health in and of itself. Studies show that exercising outdoors imparts more physiological and mental health benefits than exercise performed indoors, decreases stress, improves mood, and enhances markers of cardiovascular and metabolic health.[61,62,63] So get outdoors in the mornings, on that lunch break, or after dinner and try some exercise in the fresh air.

It's not totally clear why outdoor exercise is so effective, but there are some intriguing theories. It may be that being in a natural environment activates the parasympathetic (rest and digest) nervous system and the stress recovery response, which then improves several elements of physical health, including blood pressure, heart rate, and heart rate variability, and also positively influences mental health.[64] Or maybe the restorative qualities of outdoor environments renew and refresh our ability to pay attention, which then allows us to recover from cognitive fatigue and bolsters us against stress.[65]

It's possible that the combination of increased parasympathetic activity and decreased attentional fatigue explains why outdoor exercise has powerful physical and psychological benefits. The idea here is that when we pay attention to the details of a natural environment—the trees, leaves, sound of water, and so on—we refuel our attention system and can then pay better attention to everything else that requires our focus.

There are a lot of reasons to go green. And it's not hard to reap the benefits.

START HERE: GREEN EXERCISE IS EASY

The term *green exercise* was first introduced in 2003 to describe the synergistic effect of physical activity and being in nature. It includes activities such as trail running, hiking, gardening, and playing golf.[66]

Chronic busyness has become a barrier to exercise, but green exercise need not be time consuming or intense to be beneficial. In fact, in one study, as little as 12 to 15 minutes of forest walking resulted in positive cardiovascular and psychological health outcomes in a group of young, healthy males when compared with the same amount of time spent walking in an urban environment.[67] Even the busiest of us can spare 15 minutes once a day to get outside, whether to a local park or somewhere in the countryside.

And the good news is that this exercise need not be intense. Low-intensity gardening, for example, has been shown to have a multitude of health benefits, including reducing the risk of dementia, improving mood and self-esteem, lowering the risk for depression, increasing vigour, and decreasing cortisol.[68] And not only can your chosen activity be low intensity, but *any* activity outside seems to feel easier than doing something similar indoors. For example, people who walk outside report lower rates of perceived exertion while, paradoxically, walking faster.[69] Maybe the beauty of the outdoors is a simple distraction from feelings of effort. That's another great reason to swap the treadmill for the trail.

Want a tip to get started? Build moments of outdoor movement into your day by taking your dog for a walk, planting a garden, or stretching and meditating outdoors.

At the end of the day, all exercise is good exercise. But why not elevate your workout routine by taking it outside to enjoy the additional benefits?

A LITTLE MORE ADVANCED:
BLUE EXERCISE AND WILD SWIMMING

Simply put, wild swimming is swimming in natural bodies of water, like lakes and oceans. Which is also what *blue exercise* means: moving your body in bodies of water that are not human made. Blue mind—because of being physically close to water, like being by a lake—is a state of increased calm and wellness, better sleep, and decreased stress and anxiety.

You know the benefits of green exercise: improved physical and mental health as a result of decreased depression, stress, tension, anger, and anxiety and increased fitness and feelings of happiness. Interesting new research on the benefits of blue exercise has revealed the potential role of wild swimming in building mindfulness and resilience.[70] One case study even demonstrated that cold-water wild swimming may have therapeutic implications as a treatment for medication-resistant major depressive disorder.[71] This effect might be caused by a physiological response to cold water or by the sense of achievement and empowerment you feel when you master a challenging task.

As mentioned in an earlier section about extreme sports, the effects of extreme outdoor exercise can be cathartic. Think about the thrill of rock climbing, skydiving, or jumping off a boat to swim in deep water. The fear and the release of adrenaline during the activity stimulate the sympathetic nervous system, allowing you to release built-up aggression, anger, and tension. After the activity is over, there is a calming and stress-relieving activation of the parasympathetic nervous system, much like the effects of meditation. So next time you're angry, channel all that rage into an outdoor workout instead—in a lake, river, or ocean.

All this to say that green and blue exercise are just as good for the mind as they are for the body. And it might be easier than you think to enjoy the benefits—even if you choose more challenging physical activities.

POWER-UP #7: MOVE FOR JOY

If you're following the plot so far, you know that physical activity is one of the most effective ways to stay mentally healthy. It stimulates the growth of new neurons and enhances learning and memory. It improves creativity and boosts mood. It reduces the risk of developing depression. When we exercise, we just feel better, both physically and mentally. We are more likely to experience happiness and joy.

So why is starting and maintaining an exercise routine a huge challenge for many of us? Even when we know that exercise makes us feel good by releasing endorphins, which are hormones that can cause feelings of wellbeing, elation, and euphoria. Don't we want to be healthier and happier?

Well for one reason, not everyone gets that "runner's high" after a workout. How people respond to an exercise stimulus seems to depend on many factors, including their health, fitness level, and past experiences. There's also a question around the types of activities people choose. Do you think you are *supposed* to do something in particular—maybe train for a 10K or join a gym or take a spinning class? Are you "shoulding" yourself about the "right" way to exercise? Having an overly narrow view, perhaps influenced by a friend or family member or even a popular movement, can lead to unhappy results.

That's why some researchers suggest there isn't a universal exercise prescription: to experience the greatest psychological benefits, you should instead exercise at an intensity that "feels good."[72] Whatever feels good to you is good for you, physically and mentally. The idea is not to grind through life but to find people, places, and activities that spark joy. What do you love to do that also moves your body? That's what will make you happiest and also more likely to come back to it.

Exercise doesn't have to be running on the treadmill for an hour or counting down the minutes until your workout class is finished. Exercise can be playing with your kids in the park or meeting up with a friend to go for a bike ride. It's time to stop thinking of exercise as work and to start thinking of it as just doing something you *enjoy*.

If you've tried a few typical approaches—hiking, cycling, gardening—and nothing has quite "taken" for you, consider the two movement options outlined below.

START HERE: TRY THE JOY WORKOUT

Some exciting research suggests that the types of movement we do can impact how we feel. When we're happy, excited, and joyful, our body language reflects that. We might lift our arms or jump in the air. But it also works the other way around. When we move our bodies in a certain way, we can change the way we think and feel. In fact, research has shown that happiness and a positive emotional state can be improved simply through movement and dance.[73] What's more, even watching someone perform "happy movements" can make us feel happy and joyful.[74]

This is the idea behind the Joy Workout devised by Dr. Kelly McGonigal, a health psychologist, certified fitness instructor, lecturer at Stanford University, and author of *The Joy of Movement: How Exercise Helps Us Find Happiness, Hope, Connection, and Courage*. As she says in a 2022 *New York Times* article, there are physical movements that "don't just express a feeling of joy—research shows they can also elicit it."[75]

What are some of those movements? Here's a simple list:

- Reaching your arms up
- Swaying from side to side
- Bouncing to a beat
- Spinning with arms outstretched
- Shaking your body
- Jumping up and down
- Mimicking tossing confetti in the air

You can do these moves in any order, as quickly or as slowly as you like, as big or as small as you like, and of course you can add music that makes you feel good. Up-tempo songs seem to work well. You can also double up on the movements you really like and drop any that don't uplift you.

Some things to avoid: any movements that involve sinking or shrinking. Those types of movements evoke feelings of sadness and fear.

It's amazing that choosing specific movements, like throwing your arms up in the air, can create feelings of joy. Try making up a movement routine that works for you. Or look for Kelly McGonigal's Joy Workout.

A LITTLE MORE ADVANCED: JOIN A DANCE CLASS

With a bit more planning and commitment to a regular activity, you can find a dance-based movement class that expands on the Joy Workout in a few ways.

First, research shows that doing something with a friend, partner, or group elicits more joy than doing something alone.[76] Basically, fun is more fun with others.

Second, there is interesting research about dance music therapy, which is used to change a person's emotional state through movement and dance.[77] As with the Joy Workout, this research shows that moving your body in specific ways can regulate your emotions and increase your happiness as well as improve emotional resiliency, which is the ability to bounce back from difficulties. In addition, dance can also enhance feelings like empowerment, pride, and determination, which add to the overall positive impact of this kind of movement.

So with these two ideas in mind—being with others and moving your body rhythmically to music—you may find that a dance class provides a perfect double whammy of boosting your physical health and your emotional state: sparking both wellness and joy.

What kind of dance? That's up to you. There is no wrong answer. Again, the best activities are those that interest, engage, and inspire you. Ballroom dancing with your spouse? Absolutely. Jazz class with a friend? Definitely. Hip hop, tap, rumba, or belly dancing in a group of fellow joy generators? Go for it.

Move to Live

It's the paradox of exercise—to get energy, you have to expend some.
—JIM MCKENNA, LEEDS BECKETT UNIVERSITY

I know you've heard the expression "Use it or lose it." It turns out that "using it" is critically important where your mitochondria are concerned. It is well established that highly energetic tissues like skeletal muscle are rich in mitochondria. It is also known that physical activity increases mitogenesis, which is the creation of new mitochondria. On the other hand, chronic muscle disuse can have the opposite effect: it can lead to more damaged and dysfunctional mitochondria. This is why physical exercise is seen as an emerging tool to protect mitochondrial health.

According to the World Health Organization, globally, one in four adults and over 80% of adolescents do not meet the daily recommendations for physical activity, statistics that are particularly worrisome when considering the somber implications of muscle disuse.[78]

Dr. Jonathan Little from the University of British Columbia recently discovered that exercising for as little as 20 seconds a few times throughout the day is enough to improve cardiorespiratory fitness and overall health.[79] So if you find it hard to find time to exercise, try incorporating exercise "snacks" into your day. It can be anything: a couple of quick flights of stairs, jumping jacks, burpees, whatever gets you moving. These quick bursts of exercise improve not only your focus for the next work period but your health as well.

The key message in all of this? Try to incorporate some movement into your daily routine to keep your mitochondria in top shape. The key is consistency; use your muscles every day or lose them. To start, focus on moving a little bit every day, rather than trying to play catch-up on the weekend. And always, always focus on physical activities you enjoy, whether gentle, moderate, or intense. Your mitochondria will thank you.

ENERGIZE

HEALING, FUEL, AND POWER FOR
SUSTAINABLE HUMAN ENERGY

The energy of the mind is the essence of life.
—ARISTOTLE

Fatigue, burnout, and feeling overwhelmed are some of the biggest challenges we're facing today. Approximately 45% of the North American population is chronically fatigued, and this fatigue is associated with increased risk of developing many mental and physical diseases. In a study on fatigue in the workplace, researchers found that 65% of people with fatigue reported health-related lost productive time, and it's estimated that fatigue costs employers $136 billion annually in lost productivity.[1] Not to mention that it's hard to be happy, joyful, and excited about life when we're perpetually exhausted.

Although often used interchangeably, fatigue and burnout are a bit different. Burnout is a three-dimensional syndrome including overwhelming exhaustion, feelings of cynicism, and lack of efficacy (the ability to get things done). In addition to fatigue, burnout can make us feel overwhelmed, depleted, and numb. Exhaustion is a significant predictor of burnout and, if not addressed, can lead to burnout.[2] Like fatigue, burnout has both mental and physical consequences, such as decreased cognitive function and increased risk of developing chronic illnesses.[3,4]

This epidemic of fatigue and burnout has been exacerbated over the last few years. Many of us are feeling exhausted in ways we never did before, even if we're getting a lot of sleep and spending more time exercising. One of the reasons for this is that fatigue is not just physical—it's also mental. Recent times and events have brought about significantly more stress, anxiety, uncertainty, and a sense of being overwhelmed. We have a limited supply of mental resources, and this chronic stress drains our mental capacity, making everything harder—from exercising to concentrating at work to our ability to be present with our loved ones.

In 2021, a group of researchers looked at the impact of a high-stress situation on mental fatigue.[5] In this study, students from the University of Shanghai for Science and Technology participated in a five-day electronics design competition. The competition was important for future education and job prospects, and so the students were under significant pressure to perform well. The researchers measured mental fatigue by using an electroencephalogram (EEG) to measure brain activity. Mental fatigue became progressively worse over the course of the five days, suggesting it can accumulate during high-stress situations.

Mental fatigue also has a significant impact on physical performance. A 2017 systematic review looked at the effects of mental fatigue on exercise performance.[6] In general, studies in which participants engaged in a mentally stimulating task before exercise showed a decrease in exercise performance. However, impaired exercise performance was not due to physiological factors, such as heart rate, but rather due to a greater than normal perceived effort. In other words, participants didn't perform as well because it just *felt harder*. This is why a run feels so much harder after a stressful day at work.

Of course, it's okay to be tired and stressed in the short term. Short-term stressors are beneficial because they prime the body for future, larger stressors. But when we're not giving ourselves time to recover afterwards, we experience chronic stress, overwhelming fatigue, and, eventually, burnout. We're unable to keep up with life's demands, and even a simple task can feel daunting. However, we can break this cycle. By implementing small daily recovery tactics, we can stop this downward cycle and start performing optimally and reaching our potential.

BREAKTHROUGH IDEA: MITOHORMESIS

Did you know that mild stress promotes mitoplasticity? Agents and stimuli such as exercise, dietary caloric restriction, hypoxia (low oxygen), ischemia (low blood flow), heat exposure, and phytochemicals in fruits and vegetables induce mild cellular stress by disrupting homeostasis, increasing the demand for energy, and producing free radicals.

Counterintuitively, rather than being harmful, short-term cellular stress starts a series of signals in the cell that trigger the release of health-promoting molecules. These molecules include antioxidants, growth factors, amino acids, proteins, DNA, and RNA, all of which function to tell structures in the cell to adapt and respond by promoting detoxification, antioxidation, anti-inflammation, mitogenesis, and mitoplasticity.[7,8]

Because they promote mitochondrial growth and health, these

molecular agents have been proposed to have beneficial effects on aging and longevity as well.[9]

It is important to remember that while acute (short-term) levels of these stressors create a beneficial adaptive response, chronic stress remains detrimental to health and wellbeing.

Simply put, a little is great. A lot is not.

This process where mild environmental stressors lead to the creation of molecules that stimulate growth and adaptation in our mitochondria is called *mitohormesis*.

How Your Mitochondria Adapt to the Environment

I believe we are in the midst of a human energy crisis. As I've mentioned, chronic stress is higher than ever, leading to unprecedented levels of burnout. The best way to break this cycle is to energize our bodies at the cellular level: specifically, our mitochondria. Mitochondrial dysfunction due to abnormal levels of reactive oxygen species (ROS) and oxidative stress may be at the forefront of this chronic stress epidemic. Indeed, a study in 2008 found that work-related stress among nurses in the intensive care unit was associated with increased ROS production and that elevated markers of oxidative stress were associated with burnout.[10] Fortunately, lower levels of ROS can produce adaptive physiological disruptions that can be harnessed to our advantage and may be a potential strategy for addressing and relieving the human energy crisis. A little stress is okay, even beneficial.

Basically, too much ROS damages our mitochondria and sucks our energy. But lower levels of ROS (a little, not a lot) stimulate our bodies to adapt and improve and, in the end, generate more energy and better health.

ROS are highly reactive, oxygen-derived molecules that are mostly produced as by-products of mitochondrial electron transport, making the mitochondria especially susceptible to oxidative stress.[11] Our bodies also produce small-molecule antioxidant defences, such as superoxide dismutase and glutathione, to detoxify and attenuate the damaging effects of ROS. Oxidative stress is a state in which there is an imbalance between ROS production and removal by antioxidants, and it has profound negative physiological and cellular effects, including implications for numerous diseases. ROS and oxidative stress cause damage to mitochondrial DNA and inhibit repair machinery, cause a loss of calcium homeostasis (Ca^{2+}) and mitochondrial membrane potential, and decrease ATP and mitochondria protein production in human cells.[12] Oxidative stress also enhances the production of secondary ROS and worsens mitochondrial damage, causing a vicious cycle eventually resulting in apoptosis, which is the death of cells.[13] This vicious cycle underlies numerous metabolic, vascular, respiratory, kidney, neurological, and aging-related diseases.[14,15]

Historically, mitochondrial ROS were regarded exclusively as harmful. However, it has since been discovered that they play essential signalling roles in various physiological processes and may have adaptive functions in the human body at non-toxic levels. In other words, some amount of ROS is good and too much is bad. A process called mitohormesis describes acute (short-term) stress-producing low levels of ROS and oxidative stress as adaptive; chronic (long-term) stress that exacerbates the vicious cycle, disrupts cellular integrity, and contributes to disease states is considered maladaptive.[16] Our bodies like acute micro-stressors and use them to build strength and health—unlike chronic stressors that damage our mitochondria. Some examples of those micro-stressors are physical activity, caloric restriction, hypoxia (temporary low levels of oxygen), and temperature stress (being very hot or very cold for short bursts), as they promote health and longevity through various cellular mechanisms.[17]

Another key player in oxidative stress and mitohormesis is the inflammatory response. In fact, research shows that inflammation and ROS have a bidirectional relationship. Chronic stress causes the release of pro-inflammatory cytokines, which inhibit mitochondrial metabolism and dynamics and increase ROS production.[18] In turn, damaged mitochondria exacerbate the inflammatory response by releasing damage-associated molecular patterns (DAMPs) and ROS, activating inflammatory pathways, and causing an aberrant cycle. Conversely, studies have shown that certain types of exercise (a micro-stressor, or hormetic agent) cause the release of anti-inflammatory cytokines.[19] These anti-inflammatory mediators activate the antioxidant response element (ARE) pathway and cause the release of antioxidant enzymes, in a mitohormetic fashion.

Whew. That's how the science works. Again, the takeaway is that mild stress promotes mitochondrial growth and health, which then energizes your brain and body and protects against burnout. Read on to discover more about how a little bit of stress goes a long way.

The Challenge: The Human Energy Crisis

I've been asserting that this culture of chronic stress and burnout perpetuates the human energy crisis, leaving us feeling exhausted and unmotivated. Fortunately, there is a growing field of research focused on strategies to manage and maybe even reverse this energy crisis. Before tackling this problem, however, we need to understand the mediating role between stress and energy—which of course involves the hero of this story, our mitochondria.

Stress is defined as the physiological response of the body and brain to homeostatic disruptions—basically, forces that are pushing us out of balance. In fact, the stress response is both refereed by and targets the primary source of cellular energy, our mitochondria. When you experience stress, energy is required for neurotransmitter release and uptake, sympathetic nervous system activation, transcription and translation, and other processes that are working to re-establish homeostasis, or balance. These processes are driven by mitochondrial metabolic pathways, which break down glucose, fat, and amino acid substrates to produce ATP. Mitochondria sense the levels of these substrates and undergo fission and fusion to allostatic processes and generate signals to direct stress-induced, food-seeking behaviours. But how do environmental stress signals become coupled to these biological changes in the first place? Environmental signals like energy deficiency, hypoxia, and thermal stress are transduced into mitochondrial metabolic intermediates such as acetyl-CoA and reactive oxygen species (ROS), which travel to the nucleus and influence gene expression. Mitochondria metabolic processes then regulate the activation of transcription factors, co-activators, and epigenetic markers that mediate the expression of various genes and pathways involved in the stress response.[20]

Because stress increases the number of allostatic ATP-dependent reactions that occur in the cell at a given time, there is also increased demand for mitochondrial-dependent energy production processes. In response to this energetic demand, glucocorticoid and catecholamine stress hormones like cortisol and norepinephrine are synthesized and released from the mitochondria. These mitochondria-derived stress hormones act as mitokines to mobilize energy substrates during stress by reprogramming metabolism in various tissues depending on the energy requirements. They increase substrates to fuel mitochondria in important tissues that mediate the stress response like the heart and the brain. Reciprocally, glucocorticoids also influence the function of mitochondria. This is a process whereby low levels of glucocorticoids maintain mitochondrial membrane potential and modulate oxidation, while high levels reduce activity in the mitochondrial electron transport chain and increase ROS production.

In this way, chronic stress provokes maladaptive mitochondrial responses, further intensifying feelings of stress and burnout. It is critically important then to direct the flow of this energy toward adaptive processes that lead to positive outcomes and not maladaptive ones that result in disease and injury.

Because mitochondria are both mediated by and mediate the stress response, they are critical players in the human energy crisis. In fact, a 2020 study showed that individuals with occupational burnout had significantly lower measures of mitochondrial function when compared with controls, demonstrating the association between mitochondrial dysfunction and burnout. Consistent with the hormetic principle that small amounts of stress are adaptive, leading to positive change, a regular exercise protocol increased mitochondrial function over time in the burnout group.[21]

In practice then, inducing mild stress through various hormetic (or low-dose) methods may be an effective strategy to overcome the burnout associated with our current human energy conundrum. It seems counterintuitive, but as it turns out, to create energy, you must expend it.

STANDING ON THE SHOULDERS OF GIANTS

Dr. Marie-Helene Pelletier on Burnout

Dr. Marie-Helene Pelletier holds a Ph.D. and an MBA from the University of British Columbia and teaches leadership resilience at the UBC Sauder School of Business. She's a past director on the boards of the Canadian Psychological Association and the International Association of Applied Psychology and an active member of the Global Clinical Practice Network of the World Health Organization.

Sometimes in the resilience conversation, a lot of the focus ends up being on increasing the supply, which is a very important aspect, often one that we have most control over. There's solid research backing it up. However, you can't always win just with the supply. There are situations where the demands are going to be impossible to match, and that's very important. Otherwise, we can fool ourselves in a very unhealthy situation by continuing to try when we're trending down and need support. So considering supply and demand is very important.

Looking at both aspects, I would start with the demand side so that we personally assess it with realism. Sometimes I will ask people, "All right, start by writing down your top three stressors or demands at work. What are the three biggest things that demand your attention, that create pressure?" Then we do the same thing on the personal side.

And once we have a sense of what's going on, we can make some changes around these demands. Paying attention to the demand side helps with not thinking, "There's nothing I can change."

This process helps you to think through "Is that really the case?" It's worth keeping an open mind about this, exploring, and asking, "Do I really have to deal with all these demands all on my own?"

What most of us realize if you go through that process is that you have an opportunity to better align life with your values. And once you tap into this, a whole new world opens, and we do evolve. Things change. Revisiting is very important. And if you do then align better with your values, then you're entering the world of increased life satisfaction, increased happiness, and get more energy.

Listen to the complete interview on my podcast at https://bit.ly /DrMHPelletier.

Energy Practice

If you're not positive energy, you're negative energy.
—MARK CUBAN

Energy practice is where the rubber hits the road—where you learn how to transform your understanding of scientific concepts like mitohormesis into real-life action.

Let me start with the punchline: the energy practices I will take you through here are governed by a single principle: "A little is good and a lot is not." That's simple enough to say, isn't it? Some of the most profound things in life are simple at their core. At the same time, it's not so simple to understand why or, in many cases, how to consistently adopt the practices that follow this principle in your everyday life.

Let's go back to mitohormesis. The word describes your body's response to a certain amount—let's call it a reduced amount—of mitochondrial stress. That reduced amount of stress increases your health and vitality at the cellular level. It energizes you. Why? Because it acts as a stimulus for adaptation. It spurs your body (which includes your brain) to improve. To get better. To function at a higher level.

Let me give you a few simple examples before launching into the seven power-ups that have the potential to transform your life.

Do you get enough sleep? Most people don't. Our busy lives make it hard to get what is considered an optimal amount of sleep: between seven and nine hours per night for most adults. Less than seven hours is associated with poor health, including high blood pressure, heart disease, stroke, and depression. But guess what? More isn't better. What's called oversleeping is also associated with higher rates of mortality and disease. Both extremes—too little and too much—sap your energy and undermine your health.

The same can be said for exercise. Too little? Unhealthy. Too much? Also unhealthy. If you exercise too much, you'll feel tired, have trouble getting good sleep, have a dysregulated appetite (either too hungry or not hungry at all), suppress your immune system, trigger excessive inflammation, and so on. Again, more isn't always better.

Ditto food. Too little and you're not feeding your mitochondria adequately and generating the ATP you need for daily energy. Too much and you overwork your mitochondria, which need to process every morsel. Of course, you also gain weight and are then exposed to all the health issues that come with excess body fat, such as diabetes, heart disease, and some cancers.

You get the idea: when it comes to most things in life, it's best to avoid extremes. Maybe you've heard of the Goldilocks principle—porridge that is neither too hot nor too cold or beds that are neither too soft nor too hard.

So if the principle of "a little is good and a lot is not" is so simple, why can it be so hard to follow? Here is one thought.

We live in a culture—and especially a popular culture—that leans toward extremes. A moderate, balanced approach to life doesn't get a lot of attention. Clickbait is endemic, and by that I don't just mean those crazy headlines that lure you on to some website to earn ad revenue off your visit ("Eat this one food to live to be 100"). I'm talking more about a mindset. Our brains are attracted to novelty. That can range from wanting to buy new stuff to seeking out new experiences to wanting new solutions to old problems—even if the best solution is right in front of us. None of this is bad in itself but can be harmful in excess, if we are endlessly seeking the new. Those clickbait headlines tap into that.

Combine a desire for novelty with research that suggests our brains are hardwired for laziness—designed to conserve energy—and you can see why messages around consistency (do a certain amount of "X" daily for optimal health) and moderation (a little is good and a lot is not) aren't big sellers.[22] It's not sexy *and* it requires effort. If only we could eat one food and live to be 100.

My job is twofold: explain the science behind optimal performance and show you very practical ways you can make positive and lasting changes that allow you to live your best life.

Mitohormesis is a game-changing concept when it comes to generating the energy you need to build health, wellness, and lifespan. Providing the right stimulus for positive adaptation—some but not too much—leads to profound improvements. You want exposure to the right things in the right quantities to create the right amount of stress to generate constructive change at the cellular level.

Let's get to the energy practices that, well, I happen to think are awesome. The seven power-ups that follow are guaranteed to boost your energy and power the life of excellence you deserve.

POWER-UP #1: GO FAST TO CREATE CALM (INTERMITTENT FASTING)

Intermittent fasting is a buzzword that I'm sure you've heard in the past few years, either through social media, friends, and family or from unsolicited advice from someone at a party. Maybe you've already tried it or have considered trying it but have no idea where to start. Like any new fad, it can be very confusing and hard to decipher what is actually good for you.

But wait, how does restricting food create calm? And isn't fasting extreme—not "a little" of something that generates a positive adaptive response but rather "nothing at all"?

For the first question, fasting creates calm by resting your digestive system and helping you repair and regenerate. It also helps you rebalance the micro-organisms in your gut. Researchers at Cedars-Sinai in Los Angeles have found that removing food from your regular routine allows for the rapid expansion of a gut bacteria associated with positive health markers, such as decreased intestinal inflammation and a healthier gut barrier.[23] So the absence of food for a longer-than-typical period of time creates calm in your digestive system both by allowing it to rest and by reducing inflammation.

In response to the second question about fasting being extreme . . . well, that's a mind shift, not an actual fact. Hold in mind that fasting is not starving. It's making a deliberate decision to time your meals differently. You might delay your first meal until lunchtime. Or have two meals in a day instead of three. Or have one meal a day. Or not eat for 24 hours. There are as many ways to fast as there are folks interested in trying it.

In simple terms, intermittent fasting means having an eating plan that adds in periods of fasting or extends the period of time between meals. Changing the timing of when you eat is not an extreme event. Rather, it falls under the low-dose stress model of mitohormesis—a little food restriction goes a long way when it comes to building your health.

Here's more on the science of how that works.

Intermittent fasting is a hormetic agent because it increases antioxidant defences; promotes DNA repair, mitogenesis, and autophagy (the destruction of damaged cells); regulates protein quality control; and decreases inflammation.[24] These processes develop stress resistance within the cells in your body, much like the effects of exercise. Intermittent fasting also enhances cognition and lifespan and may have disease-modifying properties in cancer and neurodegenerative, cardiovascular, and metabolic diseases. However, as with any hormetic agent, I am talking about introducing moderate fasting into your life, not something extreme.

I've already mentioned inflammation, which is an underlying feature in chronic conditions such as diabetes, obesity, cardiovascular diseases, and depression. Intermittent fasting may have important implications in decreasing the risk of or treating these conditions. For example, evidence suggests it can help decrease the risk of cardiovascular disease, prevent the development of atherosclerosis, improve blood pressure, and increase autophagy as mentioned already, all of which are partly attributable to the reduced inflammation.[25] Indeed, a systematic review found that both caloric restriction and intermittent fasting reduce levels of the pro-inflammatory biomarker CRP, with intermittent fasting having a larger effect.[26] Both caloric restriction and intermittent fasting had greater effects when caloric intake was reduced to less than 50% of the daily recommended levels, demonstrating the importance of caloric restriction in combination with intermittent fasting.

The simplest way to reduce calories is to eliminate one of your regular meals for the day and keep the others, without making up the caloric difference. I'll talk more about that soon.

But wait, is intermittent fasting a good method for losing weight? Social media influencers and news outlets have generated considerable confusion about whether this "diet," if that's what we want to call intermittent fasting, really works for weight loss. Luckily, we can rely on the science here. A 2021 review concluded that intermittent fasting is a safe weight-loss alternative to daily caloric restriction, but with an important caveat.[27] You need to narrow your eating period and not add in your missing calories from meals you are no longer eating. With this approach, intermittent fasting is effective at restricting caloric intake without requiring you to count your calories. Basically, drop a meal from your day and eat normal amounts of food during your eating period.

Having settled that question, let me just add that another benefit of intermittent fasting is that when the body is in a fasted state, it makes a metabolic switch to rely less on glycogen, which is basically stored glucose, and draw more on fat stores for energy. This switch from burning glucose to burning fat creates ketone bodies, which can decrease cholesterol and triglyceride levels in the blood. The brain's use of ketones for fuel may even prevent age-related decreases in white matter integrity or cognitive function.[28]

Last, fasting has also been shown to increase brain-derived neurotrophic factor (BDNF), which I talked about earlier. BDNF stimulates the growth of new neurons in the brain, which is associated with improved mental capacity, the treatment of depression, and the prevention of Alzheimer's disease. Furthermore, by decreasing the amount of time we're eating throughout the day, we can shift from the sympathetic (fight or flight) to parasympathetic (rest and calm) nervous system activity and give our bodies a reset by decreasing heart rate and blood pressure and increasing heart rate variability.[29]

Want to know something else that's great about fasting? It helps us let go of the food cravings that hijack our minds. Yes, it's true. Eating less often—and sometimes eating less food overall as well—can free us from those cravings that can distract us from healthy eating or even undermine our work or home productivity. This is yet another way that fasting helps create calm in our lives.

So that's the skinny on fasting. Here are some ways to integrate it into your days.

START HERE: TRY A 16:8 OR 18:6 EATING SCHEDULE

Intermittent fasting means introducing longer periods of time into your day when you do not consume food, which includes caloric beverages that are basically food-like, such as smoothies.

Of course, we generally don't eat overnight, so that's already one fasting period in a 24-hour cycle (with "breakfast" tradition- ally breaking the fast). A 16:8 approach means not eating for 16 hours of the day and consuming all your meals in eight hours. And obviously, 18:6 means not eating for 18 hours of the day and having a six-hour window for your meals.

What does this look like? Many people who eat this way keep it simple: they have lunch and dinner. If their eating window is six hours, the timing would be around noon and 6 p.m. If it's eight hours, it's similar, just with the dinner meal possibly being later. The idea is to not consume calories before the lunch meal or after the evening meal. No snacking. Of course, you could set up any other schedule: first meal at 10 a.m. and the second at 4 p.m. or 6 p.m. Or first meal at 2 p.m. and the second at 8 p.m. or 10 p.m. What works for you will depend on your preferences and your work and social schedules.

In terms of how much to eat, there are two ways to approach this as mentioned already: you can eat all your daily calories in these two meals (making one or both of them larger than usual), or you can mix caloric restriction with your fasting. One simple way to do that is to not "eat back" what you would normally have for breakfast or after dinner.

For your beverages, drink plenty of water and non-caffeinated teas, and have coffee (if you drink coffee) as you usually would. And by the way, by *coffee* I don't mean those whipped cream and syrupy beverages. I mean black coffee or coffee with a splash or two of milk or cream.

Try a 16:8 or 18:6 eating schedule for a few weeks and see how it goes for you. If you want to combine it with caloric restriction, maybe just change your eating schedule for week one to get used to it first and then reduce calories in the following weeks.

A LITTLE MORE ADVANCED: OMAD, 5:2, OR ADF

Let me explain the acronyms. OMAD means one meal a day. A 5:2 schedule means to eat as you normally would for five days a week and then fast for two days. And ADF means alternate-day fasting, which is exactly how it sounds: eat every other day.

I won't call these extreme ways of fasting, because they're really not. But I would say they might be challenging to implement. You could start with the simpler approaches already outlined before trying one of these.

In all cases, no matter what kind of fasting you implement (with or without caloric restriction), follow the principles of healthy eating. This means limiting any food that is processed or high in sugar and reducing red meat intake, since all of these foods have been associated with higher mortality.[30] Instead, prioritize fruits and vegetables and healthy carbohydrates, fats, and proteins.

While intermittent fasting has been shown to improve physical and mental wellbeing, without major adverse effects, don't try anything more extreme (like extended fasts) before talking to a health professional.[31] For those who are pregnant or breastfeeding or who have an eating disorder or underlying condition such as diabetes or a hormonal imbalance, speak with a medical professional. Those under the age of 21 should not fast unless they are doing so for medical reasons under the supervision of a physician.

And remember, if you're going to try intermittent fasting, start small.

POWER-UP #2: GET HOT AND NOT BOTHERED (HEAT AND MINDFULNESS)

Remember our hormetic principle: a little is good and a lot is not. As it turns out, this also applies to thermal stressors. Acute exposure to hot or cold environments has fantastic health benefits, spanning a range of physiological processes and helping to energize—and calm—the body and brain.

I'm going to focus on heat here and show you how it is not only a great micro-stressor you can use to build your health but also a pathway to greater mindfulness. But first, the science of the stress, starting with heat shock proteins.

Heat shock proteins (HSPs) are a family of highly conserved proteins that respond to thermal, oxidative, and metabolic stressors and are involved in the protection against cellular stress.[32] It has been shown that repeated sauna exposure accustoms the body to heat stressors and primes the antioxidant system for future exposures via HSPs.[33] In fact, thermal stress mimics the hormetic effects of exercise, which include antioxidant activation, the release of anti-inflammatory cytokines, and protection against protein damage and aggregation. Short and frequent trips to the sauna have wonderful benefits and are an easy and healthy lifestyle practice to incorporate into your daily routine.

Heat shock proteins also play a role in mediating immune function and the cell cycle.[34] In a signalling cascade, environmental stressors such as heat activate heat shock factors, which then bind to heat shock elements and facilitate the translation of HSPs. Indeed, one study showed that six days of deep-tissue heat therapy increased levels of HSPs in a sample of healthy participants.[35]

In addition, several biomarkers of mitogenesis were elevated, and mitochondrial respiratory capacity increased by 28% from base-line, suggesting that acute recurrent heat stress induces favour-able mitochondrial adaptations and protection against cellular stress, leading to increased energy production.

This is exactly what we're looking for: just enough stress (not too much) to create positive adaptations in our cells that lead to greater energy production. Who knew that taking saunas or get-ting deep-tissue heat therapy could result in healthier cells?

Besides activating HSPs, acute heat exposure has important antioxidant and anti-inflammatory effects. One cross-sectional study of Finnish men reported that regular sauna bathing was negatively associated with serum levels of C-reactive protein, a marker of systemic inflammation.[36] Similarly, a crossover trial where participants completed 30 minutes of aerobic exercise and then followed that with either 40 minutes of seated recovery or 40 minutes of recovery in a sauna demonstrated that post-exercise heat exposure significantly reduced oxidative stress.[37]

As with other hormetic agents, however, too much heat expo-sure is dangerous at excessive levels and in special populations such as children, pregnant women, and individuals with pre-existing illnesses. Remember, we're talking about short doses of heat stress, which can have excellent energizing, antioxidant, and anti-inflammatory benefits. On the other hand, excessive expo-sure to heat can lead to heat exhaustion, stroke, malignant hyper-thermia, or hemorrhagic shock and encephalopathy syndrome.[38]

What about the mindfulness part? Another interesting fea-ture of heat therapy is that we're a little uncomfortable when we're hot. Staying in the moment is a great way to maintain our exposure, tolerate the heat, and add another benefit of practising mindfulness. When you fully attend to what's happening with all your senses, you achieve calm in your life and are much less likely to feel overwhelmed or be reactive. That develops your self-awareness, reduces your stress, and enhances your productivity. So while your cells are being slightly stressed and their health is increasing as they adapt, so too can your mind grow stronger and more resilient.

START HERE: TAKE A HOT BATH

Reaping the benefits of heat therapy can be as simple as taking a hot bath—or using a hot tub, if you have access to one. In the bath, the general idea is to set the water temperature a little above your comfort level. You want to feel hot enough to sweat. Researchers from Liverpool John Moores University have shown that an increase of only 0.6 °C in your body temperature while taking a bath three times a week for six weeks leads to improved health markers: the growth of new blood vessels, increases in insulin sensitivity, and fitness improvements.[39]

Hold in mind the general principle that thermal discomfort promotes health and then set your bath up to create those conditions for a tolerable amount of time. You can start with only 5 minutes and build up to 15 or 20 minutes. The great thing about a bath is that you can just add some cold water and then carry on with your relaxing soak once you have been sweating for long enough. Also great: bubbles. You can add some aromatherapy to your heat therapy plus the pure fun of bubbles for an overall healthful and relaxing activity.

A LITTLE MORE ADVANCED: TRY THE SAUNA

Sauna bathing induces mild hyperthermia from acute (as in short-term) exposure to temperatures ranging from 45 °C to 100 °C. As mentioned, the physiological response following a trip to the sauna is comparable to that of exercise, offering protection against various cardiovascular diseases, reducing inflammation, enhancing cognitive and mental health, increasing cardiorespiratory fitness and thermoregulation, and preserving muscle mass via mitogenesis.

You may already use a gym that has a sauna, so that's great. If not, look around and see what options are available to you. Lots of the big gym chains and some of the smaller ones offer a sauna for use. No sauna? A hot bath will work just as well.

If you're new to saunas, here are a few tips:

Drink water. Studies show that the average person loses up to 0.5 kilograms of sweat in one sauna session, so it is very important to stay hydrated.[40] Drink beforehand. When you're done, even if it's a short visit, have another glass of water or an electrolyte drink.

Start small. Try five minutes max to start out. See how you feel. Saunas can vary in temperature as well, so don't be surprised if it's hotter one day than another. Remember, sweating is healthy and normal. Feeling light-headed, sick, or dizzy is not. Over time, increase your sauna visit by a few minutes each time until you reach between 15 and 30 minutes, which is enough time for the health benefits. Also, the more often you use a sauna, the better for your health.

Take a cold shower between sessions. Allow your body to cool off for a few minutes and then take a cold shower. Alternating from heat to cold exposure has been shown to have great health benefits.[41]

Practise mindfulness. Tune in to what you're feeling through your senses—which will also help you with monitoring how well you feel. But mainly, do so to slow your mind, calm your system, and stay in the moment.

Avoid food, substances, and other drinks. Things to avoid before, during, and after a sauna: alcohol, recreational drugs, and large meals.

Practise sauna etiquette. If you've worked out beforehand, shower first, as you would before entering a swimming pool. Sit on a towel, whether nude or wearing a bathing suit. If you want to adjust the heat of the sauna, talk to others before increasing or decreasing it (also, you can move around the sauna for different temperatures—it's hotter on higher seats and cooler on lower ones). And be aware that saunas are generally quiet spaces. That shouldn't be hard for you to respect as you work on your mindfulness.

Enjoy. It should be a little uncomfortable but not excruciating to be in a sauna. That discomfort is part of the hormetic effect—just like exercise. But also like exercise, it shouldn't hurt. Experiment with designing an experience that works for you.

Saunas offer tremendous benefits, but as with any other health intervention, it may not be the right place for you if you are on certain medications, have an underlying medical condition, or are pregnant. Check with your doctor before visiting a sauna.

POWER-UP #3: CHILL OUT AND DIAL IN (COLD AND CONCENTRATION)

If you don't want to heat up, how about cooling off? Or of course, you can do both. Some people like to mix hot and cold therapy, which has been shown to have tremendous health benefits. But for our purposes here, let's just talk about the cold: what it does on the cellular level and how it can also help develop your ability to concentrate.

Similar to the heat shock response, exposure to cold activates the cold shock proteins that are essential for survival during cold acclimation.[42] Unlike heat, however, which has a blunting effect, cold exposure actually activates the parasympathetic (calming) nervous system.[43] You may find that surprising, having felt cold and not at all relaxed about it. But while initial exposure to cold activates the sympathetic nervous system, habitual exposure dampens this response and can reduce stress and anxiety in an adaptive hormetic fashion.[44] Cold exposure also improves antioxidant and anti-inflammatory capacity; increases energy expenditure, metabolism, and recovery following exercise; and enhances cognition and mental health.[45]

The benefits of cold stress are multifaceted and have mostly been studied in the context of post-exercise recovery. For example, in a study of tae kwon do athletes, cold-water immersion for 30 minutes at 10 °C following a round of tae kwon do significantly increased antioxidant enzymes in comparison with the passive recovery control group.[46] Similarly, winter swimmers were shown to have elevated total antioxidant capacity.[47]

Several studies have also found that post-exercise cooling enhances mitogenesis following endurance exercise by upregulating the upstream transcriptional regulator PGC-1α (a key regulator of energy metabolism).[48,49,50] Furthermore, cold exposure may also have implications for weight loss, as it has been shown to activate mitochondria-rich brown adipose tissue and contribute to elevated energy expenditure.[51] Likewise, a 2021 study showed that cold-water swimmers had significantly greater cold-induced brown adipose tissue and skeletal muscle thermogenesis when compared with controls, demonstrating how cold-water swimming can be used as a tool to increase energy expenditure and weight loss.[52]

As with heat stress, excessive exposure to cold temperatures can be dangerous because it lowers your core body temperature, causing cardiac stress, exhaustion, or loss of consciousness. It can also result in hypothermia, which impairs cellular metabolism, cardiovascular function, and cognition, and in extreme cases can result in death. So we're not looking for excessive or prolonged exposure to cold. We're looking for short bouts of cold temperatures that create a little stress for your system. A little is good and a lot is not.

What about your concentration? How does cold boost your productivity and ability to focus throughout the day?

We know that cold exposure robustly facilitates the release of norepinephrine into the brain and the bloodstream.[53] Norepinephrine is a neurotransmitter and hormone involved in mediating mood, attention, vigilance, and focus, and decreased norepinephrine activity is associated with impaired cognition, low energy, and poor mood. This is why cold exposure may be an effective way to increase focus, attention, and vigilance. Indeed, a randomized control trial from 2016 demonstrated that workers who took a cold shower every day for one month reported an increased sense of productivity, among other measures of wellbeing.[54] Another study that investigated the self-reported effects of practising the Wim Hof method (a combination of cold-water exposure and meditative or attention-control exercises) found that participants commonly reported positive changes in their attentional energy levels, awareness, and concentration.[55]

So next time you have a big presentation at work or need to be extra productive for the tasks at hand, try taking a short cold shower in the morning. That burst of cold stress not only creates feelings of wellness but sharpens your mental focus as well.

START HERE: TAKE A COLD SHOWER

Take advantage of temperature stress as a well-known hormetic agent by getting into a cold shower. It's the simplest way to add the benefits of cold therapy to your life.

As with adding hot temperature stress into a day, start small and then slowly build up to longer times and colder temperatures. You will slowly build tolerance to the cold and find it easier and easier to add in more time. And—believe it or not—you will even start to enjoy these wonderfully bracing moments in your day.

But at first, expect it to hurt a bit. The cold receptors in your skin are the same receptors that sense pain, so you will perceive the cold as painful. This will change over time as you maintain a cold practice.

Here's how to start: Add 30 seconds of cold at the end of your showers for one week. In week two, aim for one minute, and in week three, aim for two minutes. And so on. Eventually, you may take your entire shower cold. But if that is too extreme for you, a few minutes a day will offer the health and concentration benefits of cold therapy.

A LITTLE MORE ADVANCED:
TRY COLD-WATER IMMERSION

Cold-water immersion (CWI) has been extensively studied in the context of post-exercise recovery[56] and has been shown to decrease both intense exercise-induced inflammation and delayed-onset muscle soreness while promoting the activation of antioxidant capacity.[57] These changes represent an adaptive hormetic response that increases the body's overall antioxidant efficiency and tolerance to future stressors.[58]

A cold bath or an ice bath can be used for CWI—though few of us have easy access to a lot of ice at short notice. Outdoor CWI options include swimming in the ocean, which can be cold throughout the year depending on the location, and lake swimming in the winter. You've no doubt heard of polar bear plunges where people wade into the water in the winter months. That's the idea, only more often than once per season.

Here are some tips if you would like to try CWI.

Ease into it. The effects of CWI depend on the temperature of the water and the time spent submerged. Most studies report positive effects after 5 to 20 minutes in water at 10 to 15 °C.[59] As mentioned already, if you are new to CWI you can start with a few minutes of cold shower time and work your way up. If you're feeling brave, try jumping in a cold lake or pond. Take cold-water showers or ice baths for 30 days at home before trying outdoor CWI in order to allow your body to become accustomed to the physiological response. Be cautious when you are cold swimming outdoors, as even a 20-second plunge into water at 4 °C has been shown to significantly increase norepinephrine levels.[60]

Be mindful of the risk. While a cold shower is much safer and the temperature can be easily regulated, wild swimming in a cold lake or pond may have benefits above and beyond that of a shower. Outdoor swimming can be dangerous, however, as excessive exposure to cold water induces cardiac stress and hyperventilation. Hypothermia occurs quickly after submersion in water at 4 °C or less.[61] Always bring a buddy for supervision.

Get warm as quickly as possible. The Outdoor Swimming Society recommends drying yourself immediately, dressing in dry and warm layers, bringing a hat and gloves, drinking a warm beverage, and eating a snack immediately following a cold-water swimming session.[62] Your body temperature continues to drop even after exiting the water, so it is important to warm up in a gradual and safe manner

As with heat therapy, there can be dangers for some people. Avoid CWI if you are immunocompromised, have a heart condition or high blood pressure, have recently recovered from an illness or hospitalization, or are otherwise ill.

POWER-UP #4: LIGHT UP YOUR LIFE (SUNLIGHT AND ENERGY)

Sunlight has loads of health benefits and is mitohormetic as well, meaning sun exposure generates a low-level stress response that leads to positive adaptations at the cellular level.

But wait, isn't this the same sun that emits the ultraviolet (UV) radiation that can cause skin cancer? Aren't we supposed to avoid the sun to protect our skin and our health?

Well, yes and no. Remember our hormetic principle: a little is good and a lot is not. We don't want to avoid sunlight entirely because it offers so many benefits, including an increase in overall energy. But we also don't want to bake ourselves into ill health. Let me explain further to set the scene for your light needs and energy outcomes.

I'm guessing you've heard about the benefits of vitamin D—and sunlight is our best source of it. In scientific terms, vitamin D is a critical mediator of cellular oxidative stress, systemic inflammation, and mitochondrial respiration.[63] The activated form of vitamin D, calcitriol, does so by activating gene transcription, cellular response elements, and second-messenger signalling cascades. Indeed, vitamin D deficiency is associated with increased oxidative stress, impaired mitochondrial function, and systemic inflammation, and it increases the incidence and severity of various metabolic disorders, including type 2 diabetes, autoimmune diseases, hypertension, and more.

Of course, as with all hormetic agents, too much sunlight is not healthy. For example, it suppresses the immune system, causing autoimmune diseases and tumorigenesis, so what I am talking about here is frequent but moderate sunlight exposure and not letting your skin burn.[64]

Here's more good news about vitamin D. It is necessary for numerous physiological processes such as the maintenance of calcium and phosphate homeostasis and bone mineralization; bone growth and remodelling; the regulation of inflammation and oxidative stress; cell growth, proliferation, and apoptosis; neuromuscular function; and glucose metabolism.[65] It can also be protective against autoimmune diseases, cancer, osteoporosis, bone fractures, muscle weakness, cognitive dysfunction, depression, hypertension, metabolic syndrome, obesity, and diabetes.[66] Whew. That's quite a list.

There are dietary sources of vitamin D, such as fatty fish, fish liver oils, egg yolks, and milk products that are fortified. However, adequate levels of the vitamin cannot be obtained from the diet alone.[67] The best natural source of vitamin D is sunlight, which is produced after the skin is exposed to UV radiation. Cholecalciferol (vitamin D_3 produced by the sun) is a prohormone and must be transformed into its biologically active form (calcitriol) by hydroxylation reactions in the liver and kidney. Upon activation, calcitriol binds to the vitamin D receptor, triggering gene transcription, cellular response elements, and second-messenger signalling cascades.[68]

How well our bodies generate vitamin D is affected by geographical factors including climate, altitude, weather, season, latitude, and pollution, as well as individual differences such as skin colour, melanin, and genetics. For example, some places have fewer daylight hours than others. A little village called Rjukan in Norway receives no sunlight for six months of the year. Compare that with the town of Yuma in Arizona, which is known to be the sunniest place on Earth, with up to 13 hours of sunlight every day in the summer months.

Sunlight also has many other benefits in addition to vitamin D production. For example, modest levels of UV radiation induce the synthesis of nitric oxide, which reduces hypertension, improves cardiovascular health, and protects against oxidative stress and inflammation. UV radiation has also been shown to increase the expression of the anti-inflammatory, anti-apoptotic, anti-proliferative, and antioxidant-involved gene heme oxygenase-1, which protects your cells from injury and oxidative stress and is protective against the autoimmune disorder multiple sclerosis.[69] Novel quantum physics research demonstrates an emerging role for sunlight and mitochondrial function by showing that photons directly affect mitochondria by modulating the viscosity of the mitochondrial-bound water layer and regulating the activity of ATP synthase.[70,71] Finally, sunlight is remarkable for its effects on mood and mental health. It has been shown to cause the release of serotonin, significantly improving mood and relieving symptoms of several psychiatric mood and anxiety disorders.[72]

But as mentioned already, as with all hormetic agents, too much sunlight exposure can be detrimental. Excessive sunlight-induced nitric oxide production, for example, can cause edema, inflammation, and immune suppression, which can lead to the development of autoimmune diseases and tumorigenesis.[73] Furthermore, as a carcinogen, the main cause of skin cancer is UV radiation, which activates reactive oxygen species that target and damage DNA.[74] Fortunately, there are easy ways to protect yourself against the damaging effects of the sun.

Let's take full advantage of this natural source of health and energy while minimizing its dangers. Step one: get up, get outside, leave your fake light (phone) at home, and get real light into your eyes and brain.

START HERE: GET OUTSIDE AND PRACTISE SUNBATHING

No, I'm not talking about slathering baby oil on your skin and roasting on a beach all day. Instead, follow these practices to reap all the health and energy rewards of glorious sunlight.

How much time should I spend in the sun? It is thought that 5 to 15 minutes of sunscreen-free sunlight exposure at around midday, several times a week, is sufficient for your body to produce enough vitamin D without getting a sunburn.[75] According to the Multiple Sclerosis Society of Canada, vitamin D is optimally synthesized from sunlight at midday during the spring and summer months in Canada when the UV index is greater than 3.

Does sunscreen prevent vitamin D production? It is thought that sunscreen may interfere with sunlight-induced vitamin D production, but research demonstrates that concerns about vitamin D should not negate those of skin cancer.[76] According to a 2019 literature review, the risk of sunscreen inhibiting vitamin D production or causing vitamin D deficiency is low, so don't skip the sunscreen if you're going outside for more than 15 minutes.

What SPF should I wear? Sunscreen with a sun protection factor (SPF) of 15 or higher has been shown to reduce the risk of melanoma, carcinoma, and premature skin aging.[77] SPF 30 sunscreen filters out 97% of UV rays that reach the skin, while SPF 50 filters out 98%, making SPF 30 a great choice.

What kind of sunscreen should I wear? Mineral sunscreens containing UV filters such as zinc oxide and titanium dioxide work by reflecting or refracting UV radiation off the skin and have been established as safe and effective.[78] Chemical sunscreens, on the other hand, which absorb UV radiation, are more available and may confer better protection. However, they have come under some scrutiny regarding their safety, though there is no clear evidence that they cause direct harm. This remains a subject of debate, with many people opting to use mineral sunscreen instead.

That's it. Get outside and practise sun safety at the same time. You'll boost your mood, build your health, and replenish your energy stores.

A LITTLE MORE ADVANCED:
RESPECT THE NEED FOR DARKNESS

Here I am going to advocate for adding an extra element to your daily sunshine bathing that will make you even more energized and productive. I want to call out what I believe to be a serious issue in today's world, which is that, instead of waking and sleeping with the sun's cycle, we are constantly exposed to artificial light and screens all day long.

This is an issue because when light hits your eyes, it sends a signal to your brain that it's daytime and to stop producing melatonin, the hormone that makes you feel sleepy, with the blue light from screens particularly bad. One of the most effective ways to fall asleep quickly (and have a restful sleep) is to avoid exposing your eyes to bright light within the hour before you'd like to be asleep. I call this "defending your last hour." Have an alarm set to go off every night one hour before you'd like to be asleep. At this point, put away devices and start winding down your body and brain for a deep and restful sleep.

Here are tactics you can use.

First, be intentional about devices and exposure to light. People tend to think that devices emit a steady stream of light, but they actually flash at us so fast we can't see it happening. Computers, tablets, and phones operate at 30 to 60 frames per second. Televisions are 120 to 240 frames per second.

Conversely, a nightlight operates on AC current, which is a sine wave. It is not flashing at you. It's a constant flow of light, which you can turn down to emit as little light as possible.

In our home, my family creates a digital sunset every evening. All of our lights are on dimmer switches. Around six o'clock, I'll walk around and dim the lights. My son, Adam, starts walking into walls. We eventually just pick him up and throw him into bed. It's awesome. In our bedroom, we have dim nightlights, and we don't take devices to bed.

When you wake up in the morning, feel free to zap your brain with light. Blue light is good for you in the morning. But in the evenings, limit light exposure.

Second, keep your room dark at night. Once you're away from screens and have completed your before-bed routine, focus on reducing all the light in your bedroom from every source. Our eyes are very sensitive to light signals and may interpret that alarm clock light, hallway light, and, of course, early morning light as commands to "wake up." Having your eyes closed doesn't protect you from seeing light, which is why having light in your surroundings is known to disrupt sleep. And you may not make the connection, because your sleep can be disrupted without your fully waking up. You may spend less time in the deeper, more restorative sleep stages and wonder why you feel draggy during the day despite logging eight hours.

The key takeaway here is that respecting the incredible power of sunlight goes hand in hand with respecting the power of darkness. Get your sunshine . . . and then turn off all the lights and drop those blackout shades. Together, those two practices will rocket-boost your energy.

POWER-UP #5: PSYCH UP AND CALM DOWN (REST AND PERFORM)

Flow states and peak performance go hand in hand. Remember that flow is an optimal psychological state during which you are completely immersed in an activity, totally focused, highly productive, and often unaware of the passage of time. This is when you're at your best, which is why athletes often report that their peak performances are characterized by flow factors.

That connection makes sense, especially since the American Psychological Association defines peak performance as the "performance of a task at the optimum level of an individual's physical abilities, mental capabilities or both."[79] Peak performance is when you are at a superior level of functioning: stronger, quicker, and more creative, productive, and efficient. That's why athletes, artists, business leaders, musicians, and so on may define peak performance in different ways. You may have your own definition as well.

Peak performance is most extensively studied in athletes and has repeatedly been defined as feeling effortless, automatic, and calm, with minimal to no distractions or conscious thoughts during the performance.[80] That overlaps a lot with flow. The peak performance you strive for in your life may also be something physical, like a personal best on the tennis court or in the city marathon. Or it may be more creative, expressed on a canvas or keyboard. Or it may be related to your work performance, perhaps bringing a new project to life or presenting to a room full of colleagues.

Whatever peak performance means to you, it shares something with everyone else's: it's influenced by our mitochondria. In other words, it's heavily dependent on energy processes.

Besides their obvious physical performance-enhancing effects, mitochondria play a critical role in brain function and cognition. As I've explained, our brains consume about 20% of our bodies' energy. That amount of energy consumption makes the brain especially vulnerable to mitochondrial dysfunction. The survival of our neurons is dependent on mitochondrial function, and healthy mitochondria make our brains function better, allowing us to cultivate the sharp focus, concentration, and energy required for peak performance. Because of the psychological nature of peak performance, the importance of your mitochondria truly cannot be overstated.

So how can you achieve peak performance when you're under pressure or doing something important to you? Here are some suggestions.

START HERE: PSYCH UP

Just as athletes must calm their nerves to curb anxiety before a big competition, it is equally important that they get themselves psyched up or "in the zone." According to the Yerkes-Dodson law, there is an optimal level of arousal that correlates to heightened performance, while both over- and under-arousal impair performance.[81] So how do athletes obtain this optimal level? And how can you apply it to your own performance-based goals?

Eliminate external distractions. Multitasking is easier and more tempting than ever with the ubiquitous nature of handheld technologies and constant media distractions. A literature review investigating the effects of media multitasking and academic performance found that using two or more media at the same time, such as texting, emailing, or browsing social media, negatively interfered with working memory and attention in an academic setting.[82] This interference reduced the efficiency, GPA, test performance, recall, self-regulation, and note-taking abilities of students. So next time you're doing an activity that is important to you, put away your smart phone and eliminate as many other external distractions as you can to encourage peak performance.

Listen to music. According to exercise physiologist Costas Karageorghis, music can both psych us up (usually higher tempo, 120–130 beats per minute) or calm us down (usually lower tempo, 70–90 beats per minute). Music shifts us into an optimal psychological state and influences blood pressure and heart rate, which are both necessary for optimal performance. For example, Canadian aerial skier Marion Thénault has both "Whatever It Takes" by Imagine Dragons (135 beats per minute) and the slower hip hop song "Hall of Fame" by The Script featuring Will.i.am on her pre-competition playlist.[83] Music is very individualized when it comes to performance, so experiment and find something that works for you.

Move your body. Movement increases your heart rate and gets your blood flowing. You'll often see athletes pacing, jogging, or jumping up and down before a race to get themselves amped up. For example, as a part of his pre-race routine, swimming legend Michael Phelps used to swing his arms and repeatedly slap himself. These psych-up techniques work by increasing intensity and arousal, subsequently improving performance.[84]

Use high-energy positive self-talk. Self-talk is one of the most powerful tools in our psychological toolbox. Repeating high-energy phrases or positive mantras, such as "I can win this" or "Attack" keeps us motivated and in a state of high energy and focus, while negative self-talk such as "There is no way I can win" has the opposite effect. For example, Bill Rodgers, former marathon world record holder, used the mantra "Relentless" to spur himself on during his gruelling races and went on to become one of the greatest distance runners of the 1970s and '80s.[85]

A LITTLE MORE ADVANCED: CALM DOWN

Hang on, how is calming down a more advanced technique for achieving peak performance than psyching up? That doesn't make sense. Except it does, and here's why: In the face of launching into a performance where you want to be your best, where you want to reach your peak, where you want to rock the world (and yourself), there's nothing harder than achieving a state of mental and emotional calm. And, in some ways, nothing more critical.

Consider professional athletes again. With the whole world watching them closely, they deal with an immense amount of pressure to perform at their best each and every time they step up to compete. Because of this, they must develop strategies to relax and manage their anxiety so that they can perform at this elite level. One way they do that is to decrease their training load leading up to a big event, which paradoxically helps increase their performance.

Athletes rely on what's called tapering to achieve peak performance at key moments. The principle is that fatigue decreases faster than fitness. Although elite athletes have incredible fitness, during a high training period their performance suffers because of physical and mental fatigue. However, leading up to a big event, when training load is reduced, they are able to decrease fatigue while maintaining their high fitness level. With proper timing, they can maximize the gap between fitness and fatigue and set themselves up to achieve a peak performance when it matters most.

While tapering is usually a term reserved for reducing training load in athletes, the principle can be applied to all of us. If we don't give ourselves sufficient time to recover, we become exhausted, burned out, and stressed, and our performance suffers. But if we allow ourselves to have proper rest—both physically and mentally—we are able to amplify our performance.

Athletes start to gradually decrease their training load as much as three weeks leading up to an event. However, you can start to boost your energy and mood after just one day of intentional rest. Apply some of these common relaxation tips from the professional athletes themselves to achieve your peak performance.

Breathe. By now, you know all about deep breathing exercises, which work by slowing your heart rate and stimulating the vagus nerve of the parasympathetic nervous system, triggering a relaxing and stress-relieving response. Olympic cyclist Laura Kenny worked with psychologists to implement a breathing-based systematic muscle relaxation technique to optimize her performance and reduce anxiety at the 2016 Rio Games.

Release tension. Your physical responses to stress are the easiest to recognize. When stress levels rise, your breathing becomes shallow, and you might clench your jaw or tense your muscles. Notice whether this happens and take a moment to consciously relax your face, shoulders, hands, stomach muscles, back, legs, and feet. Beginning at your head and working down, scan your body and release tension each time you exhale.

Visualize. As the most decorated Olympian of all time with 28 medals, swimmer Michael Phelps used visualization to deal with the intense pressure by imagining every possible scenario before a race and exactly how he would deal with it. By visualizing both the expected and the unexpected, Phelps prepared himself for anything, so that when he was actually faced with a particular situation, it did not feel foreign and he was better able to manage his stress and nerves. In this way, visualization is an effective strategy to boost both motivation and performance while calming your nerves.

Focus on the process, not the outcome. Refocusing on the process of the performance rather than the outcome has been the most important element of peak performance that I have been teaching for the last few years. Research backs this approach up. Mastery-oriented individuals are more intrinsically motivated, are more interested in the task at hand, are more likely to complete a task for its own sake, and will persist for longer. Because of this, mastery-oriented individuals are also much more likely to experience flow and peak performance. So think less about the outcome and enjoy the process instead.

Adopt a ritual. Research shows that rituals help us buffer against anxiety and uncertainty to guide goal-directed performance. An excellent example of this is two-time Olympic slopestyle gold medallist Jamie Anderson. Anderson credits her calm, confident, and focused demeanour at the Olympics in 2014 to her pre-race ritual based around calming meditation.

Rest, relax, and calm yourself before the big event, whether that means taking a break from practising (a speech or presentation or musical piece) or taking some pre-performance time to breathe, visualize, and so on. These calming techniques lead to greater adaptation, greater reserves of strength and energy, and better performance—possibly even peak performance.

POWER-UP #6: FUEL UP THE HEALTH TANK (ANTIOXIDANT NUTRITION)

While small amounts of oxidative stress may have beneficial hormetic effects, chronic oxidative stress is detrimental to our cells and is an underlying factor in chronic disease.[86] As with inflammation, many antioxidant diets have been developed over the years, such as the DASH diet, which has been shown to significantly increase levels of the antioxidant glutathione (GSH) and decrease levels of malondialdehyde (MDA), a marker of oxidative stress.[87] Antioxidant diets are composed of plant-based foods and other whole foods. Pro-oxidant diets, on the other hand, include high-fat, -carbohydrate, and -protein foods that increase oxidative stress by reducing antioxidant status and increasing lipid peroxidation and protein carbonylation.

Phenolic compounds are natural primary antioxidants found in a variety of health foods such as berries, spinach, beans, oats, ginger, quinoa, and more.[88] Studies show that these superfoods have important antioxidant, anti-inflammatory, antimicrobial, anti-tumour/cancer, cardioprotective, neuroprotective, and anti-diabetic effects. Modify your diet by substituting highly processed, sugary foods with these whole, unprocessed superfoods.

START HERE: HEALTHY FATS, VITAMINS, AND MINERALS

Here are a few simple ways you can fuel up for health and healing and, therefore, for optimal energy.

Healthy fats. Along with their anti-inflammatory role, omega-3 PUFAs (polyunsaturated fatty acids) play a critical role in our cells' ability to deal with stressors. The omega-3 fatty acids are ALA (alpha-linolenic acid), EPA (eicosapentaenoic acid), and DHA (docosahexaenoic acid). ALA scavenges free radicals and grabs or binds with toxic metals, so it plays a role in alleviating various diseases involving oxidative stress such as diabetes, atherosclerosis, heart diseases, cataracts, and neurodegenerative diseases.[89] It also has the unique ability to directly bind to and recycle endogenous GSH (which protects cells against injury), as well as mimic the glucose-uptake actions of insulin, inhibit pro-inflammatory pathways, and increase mitogenesis. Similarly, EPA and DHA have been shown to enhance total antioxidant capacity, increase mitochondrial respiratory function, enhance mitogenesis, and improve the sensitivity of adenosine diphosphate (an energy molecule).[90,91] All of this means your mitochondria become healthier and more powerful, thus increasing your strength and resilience.

Eat dietary sources of ALA, EPA, and DHA such as flaxseed and canola oils, chia seeds, walnuts, oysters, and fish such as salmon, tuna, and mackerel.

Limit unhealthy saturated fats that increase both oxidative stress and inflammation and are found in foods such as butter, cheese, meat products, and fast food, as well as refined carbohydrates including white pasta, soft drinks, white bread, and many breakfast cereals.[92,93]

Vitamins and minerals. Nicotinamide (NAD), also known as niacin or vitamin B_3, is a critical precursor to NADH, a key component of the electron transport chain, and has excellent antioxidant properties. Fish, poultry, whole grains, and fresh foods are rich in niacin. NAD deficiencies reduce mitochondrial membrane potential, glycolysis, and ATP production and increase inflammation. The other B vitamins such as thiamin (B_1), riboflavin (B_2), pantothenic acid (B_5), pyridoxal (B_6), biotin (B_7), folate (B_9), and cobalamin (B_{12}) also play a role in mitochondrial energy metabolism and have varying antioxidant roles. Vitamin C, vitamin E, and carotenoids (provitamin A) are also potent antioxidant vitamins found mostly in fruits, vegetables, nuts and seeds, and vegetable oils.[94] Sweet potato, a staple of the Okinawa diet, is an excellent source of the antioxidant vitamins A and C, as well as the B vitamins.

The trace minerals zinc and selenium also have antioxidant effects. Zinc reduces oxidative stress by facilitating antioxidant enzyme production and enzyme catalysis, participates in lipid and glucose metabolism, and acts as a cellular signalling factor to reduce levels of inflammatory cytokines; zinc can be found in oysters, beef, crab, beans, and cashews.[95] Selenium, found in Brazil nuts, tuna, halibut, and sardines, protects against ROS-mediated damage. Deficiencies in selenium cause oxidative stress.

Eat foods rich in vitamins and trace elements such as seafoods, legumes, carrots, oranges, brown rice, and lentils.

A LITTLE MORE ADVANCED: BIOACTIVE SUBSTANCES

If you enjoy digging deeper into the science of nutrition and energy, read on. There's always more to learn—and more we can do—about optimizing our fuel sources to optimize our lives.

Phytochemicals. Phytochemicals act as important antioxidants and induce hormesis—the adaptive stress-resistant process we are seeking.[96] The two most significant antioxidant-contributing phytochemicals found in plants and foods are polyphenols and carotenoids.[97] These phytochemicals are potent free-radical scavengers and anti-inflammatory agents. Polyphenols are the most prevalent natural antioxidants found in the human diet and consist of five different classes: flavonoids, tannins, coumarins, stilbenes, and phenolic acids, which can be found in wine, green tea, coffee, grapes, cherries, and chocolate.[98] Carotenoids, such as alpha and beta carotene, lutein, lycopene, and cryptoxanthin, are responsible for the orange, yellow, and red colours of different foods and are found in vegetables and fruits including sweet potato, spinach, carrots, bell peppers, beans, and pumpkin.

Eat a colourful diet rich in phytochemicals, including squash, tomatoes, broccoli, berries, whole grains, walnuts, and apples.

Other bioactive substances: Co-enzyme Q10 (CoQ10) is a fat-soluble nutrient that forms an important component of the inner mitochondrial membrane electron transport chain and acts as a powerful antioxidant.[99] It is produced by the body but can also be obtained from dietary sources such as poultry, eggs, fatty fish, nuts, and organ meats. CoQ10 prevents oxidative stress, protects against mitochondrial damage, has anti-inflammatory properties, and participates in metabolic pathways, making it an excellent antioxidant fuel for your mitochondria.[100,101]

Pyrroloquinoline quinone (PQQ) is a vitamin-like compound that can be found in foods such as spinach, soybeans, kiwi, green tea, and human breast milk.[102] It is a potent antioxidant, acts as a co-factor for many important enzymes, and targets genes involved in fatty acid metabolism and mitochondrial function, enhancing mitochondrial gene expression, content, oxidation, and biogenesis while also reducing inflammation, ischemia, and lipotoxicity.[103]

Finally, the most important antioxidant, GSH, is both produced by the cell and obtained in the diet from avocados, asparagus, okra, and spinach.[104] Dietary GSH is poorly absorbed, however, so methods to boost GSH levels include consumption of vitamin C, ALA, whey protein, foods rich in selenium such as shellfish, pork, and eggs, and N-acetylcysteine, which is primarily found in onion. These alternative sources increase endogenous GSH and have varying antioxidant effects.

Eat foods rich in endogenous antioxidants—that is, antioxidants created by your own metabolism—such as green peppers, soy products, salmon, mackerel, kale, sweet potatoes, and broccoli.

Hold the key principle in mind: whole, fresh foods are the best and healthiest choices for generating energy in your system. Go for variety and stay away (as much as possible) from foods (and food-like substances) created in factories and offered by fast-food outlets. As they say, mainly shop the outer edges of your supermarket and avoid most of what's offered in aisle after aisle of packaged foods.

POWER-UP #7: GIVE YOUR ENERGY AWAY TO GET MORE BACK (GRATITUDE AND ALTRUISM)

How is it possible to get back more than you give away? If you give away money, you have less money. If you give away goods, you have fewer goods. If you give away time, you have reduced availability.

But human emotional energy systems—which are tied to our physiological energy systems—don't have to work that way. Sometimes, giving can earn big rewards, including energy rewards. Think about giving someone love and being loved in return. Or giving your children or your pets your time and attention. Or helping an elderly neighbour with their lawn or shopping. There are many ways that we enjoy tremendous "compensation" when we give something of ourselves to others or to causes we believe in or even just out to the universe.

That's how gratitude works. Researchers define gratitude as "the appreciation of what is valuable and meaningful to oneself; it is a general state of thankfulness and/or appreciation."[105] The fundamental building blocks of gratitude consist of appreciating others, focusing on what you have, feeling awe toward beauty, focusing on positives, appreciating that life is short, and making positive social comparisons.

As it turns out, gratitude is a simple yet effective way to promote physical and emotional health and wellbeing. For example, gratitude interventions have been shown to produce long-lasting reductions in perceived stress, depression, fatigue, and feelings of hopelessness while increasing feelings of optimism, perceived control over illness, and sleep quality.[106] Gratitude promotes positive feelings and emotions such as happiness, and it also produces measurable physical changes such as reduced blood pressure, levels of cortisol, inflammation, and neurodegeneration, as well as increased heart rate variability. Gratitude is also linked with a lower risk of depression, anxiety, and substance use disorders.

But how is all this possible? According to Emiliana Simon-Thomas, director of the University of California Berkeley's Greater Good Science Center, gratitude promotes feelings of connectedness, trust, safety, and optimism, facilitating physical and mental resilience.[107] Furthermore, our mitochondria have been shown to respond to fluctuations in mood, and positive mood states are associated with greater mitochondrial health.[108] As we know, healthy mitochondria build our overall health and energize us and may thus be a mediating factor in the relationship between gratitude and health and wellbeing.[109]

Beyond gratitude, also consider altruism. Simply put, altruism can be defined as a cooperative, generous, or kind behaviour that is aimed at helping others in need but that is of no specific benefit to you and may even come at a cost or sacrifice.[110] Altruistic behaviours can be as simple as holding the door for someone or as involved as donating a kidney to a stranger. A philosophy called effective altruism is aimed at encouraging as much good as possible considering the finite resources, time, and abilities individuals possess.[111] It is a way of optimizing the contributions and differences you can make in the world.

Altruism is a natural human tendency. One study showed that

even babies show altruism and will spontaneously hand over a piece of tasty fruit to a stranger, even when they are hungry.[112] Research shows that some individuals tend to be more altruistic than others, which may be associated with structural brain differences or environmental influences such as religious affiliation or socio-economic status.[113] Interestingly, altruism can be mapped in the brain, with functional magnetic resonance imaging studies showing altered activity during altruistic behaviours in the regions associated with mentalizing, emotional salience, and reward processing, including the medial prefrontal cortex, ventral tegmental area, and amygdala.[114]

Sociobiological research suggests that altruism functions not only at the level of the organism but also at the level of genes to influence natural selection and is thus an evolutionary-supported program.[115] Therefore, it is not too far-fetched to imagine it is connected to important cellular physiological processes. In fact, Dr. Theoharis Theoharides, professor of pharmacology and immunology at Tufts University, suggests that altruism protects our microbiome health and keeps us alive and well.[116]

Additionally, altruistic behaviour may be associated with mitochondrial cooperativity, as research shows that at the cellular level, mitochondria share several important social processes with humans, including functional interdependence, which is a feature of altruism and cooperativity among social groups.[117] In this respect, mitochondria can be considered as social organelles, with both their structure and function dependent on social processes.[118] Reciprocally, they may influence social behaviours such as altruism and health through molecular, cellular, organellar, and organismal processes.[119]

Although altruism may come at a small personal cost, research shows that in the long term, unselfish individuals are happier, have better physical and mental health, have lower rates of mortality, are less stressed, and find life to be more meaningful.[120,121] One study demonstrated that altruism is immediately intrinsically rewarding by showing that participants who performed altruistic behaviours in a laboratory perceived the surrounding ambient environment as warmer.[122] Interestingly, research demonstrates that practising altruism can even relieve physical pain in unpleasant situations, a finding associated with altered brain activity in the insula and ventromedial prefrontal cortex.[123] Researchers call these long-term payoffs reciprocal altruism, referring to the ways in which helping others can help you as well.

Let's focus on how you can integrate these two practices—gratitude and altruism—into your life and benefit from the giving and getting energy upcharge.

START HERE: PRACTISE GRATITUDE

Now that you know the benefits, here are some simple ways to facilitate resilience and wellbeing by incorporating simple gratitude practices into your daily routine.

Keep a gratitude journal. At the end of every day, take five minutes to write out five reasons why you are grateful in your journal. Examples include "I am grateful for my family," "I am grateful that I am in good health when many others are not," "I am grateful that my presentation went well today at work." To mix it up a little, make a gratitude jar or try a gratitude journalling app. The key with these methods is consistency, so do it every day.

Communicate your gratitude to others. Write a letter to your friend, FaceTime your parents, or send a text to your sibling and tell them why you appreciate them. Make it a habit to thank at least one person every day. Leave a sticky note on a co-worker's desk, thank them in an email, or tell them in person. These are simple ways to build gratitude and appreciate those in your life, the connections you have with them, and how they have helped you.

Get outside. Remember awe walks? One of the fundamental components of gratitude is appreciating beauty, and what better way to realize this beauty than by immersing yourself in nature. Go for a 15-minute nature walk, take your lunch break outside, or walk your dog. Not only will you find gratitude in the beauty of nature, but you'll also get all the great benefits of green exercise.

Slow down. Meditation is a great way to slow down and appreciate the brevity of life. It allows us to ground ourselves in the present moment and focus our attention and awareness. The benefits of gratitude meditation, a positive psychological practice, overlap with those of both gratitude and meditative practices to promote overall health and wellbeing. Take 10 minutes out of your day to follow along with a guided gratitude meditation video of your choice.

Reframe negative situations. Think about how you can find the silver lining in moments of hardship. Hardship makes us tougher and stronger humans and builds resiliency and gratitude. Next time you face a hardship, focus on how you can avoid that situation in the future or the valuable lessons you may have learned.

Live simply. Walk to the grocery store instead of taking your car, or turn off the air conditioning in your room for a few nights. The next time you indulge in these creature comforts, you'll appreciate them so much more. Live simply and you'll be that much more appreciative of the things you take for granted in your life.

A LITTLE MORE ADVANCED: PRACTISE ALTRUISM

Here are some simple and easy ways you can start upon the path to becoming an effective altruist.

Help one person every day. Psychology tells us that those who perform one act of kindness every day feel happier after just six weeks.[124] Start small, like giving the employee at the drive-through a nice tip, or buying a sandwich and drink for someone in need, or topping up somebody's parking metre. Make these gratifying exercises a part of your daily routine.

Do what you're good at. The main facet of effective altruism is the practice of using your unique talents and passions to make the greatest difference possible. Research demonstrates that we experience the greatest benefits and can do the greatest amount of good when we are doing something we excel at or are passionate about.[125] Projects of passion are easier and more motivating than those you are less experienced in or unfamiliar with. Instead of volunteering for a charity or cause you have never heard of, draw on your existing pool of skills and talents and use them to your advantage.

Encourage others. Humans can accomplish so much more by making altruism a group effort. Educate others on the causes you are passionate about, or encourage them to advocate for causes they identify with. Lead by example and inspire others to do the same.

Discover the ways in which you're already giving. Keep a journal, and at the end of each week, write down all the ways in which you have helped others. You might be surprised to find how much you're already doing, and how much small gestures can help others. Furthermore, taking time to reflect allows you to discover ways in which others have helped you—and find ways to thank them.

Finally, remember that we're all in this together. One of the most important hurdles to overcome on your path to altruism is group differences. As humans, we feel more obligated to help members of our so-called in-group and less so for our out-group.[126] But we can easily modify who belongs to our in-group. The key is to remember that all humans share a common experience and we are all in this together.

Energy for Life

We live as ripples of energy in the vast ocean of energy.
—Deepak Chopra

In the midst of the COVID-19 pandemic, I called my dear friend Dr. James Rouse. I needed to talk about nutrition and my approach to eating.

I normally travel a lot. Which means I am on the go constantly. It's great—I love my work—but it's hard to be away from my family so often. But during COVID I was home all the time. I was not travelling at all. So I was not walking through the airport, hauling bags, climbing stairs, speaking on stages, or doing any of the other physical activities I do on a daily basis that I take for granted. My normal way of eating wasn't working for me. I was feeling lethargic. Food that normally fuels me was making me tired. Perhaps you noticed that the fridge was too accessible while we were all working at the kitchen table for a couple of years?

When I talked to Dr. Rouse, whom I consider to be the world's leading expert on healthy eating and positive mindset, he suggested a subtle shift in my thinking around nutrition. As an athlete, coach, and highly active public speaker, I had thought of my food as fuel. Now I needed to shift to thinking of my nutrition as healing. I needed to consider what I ate as my daily medicine for exponential health and wellbeing.

I think that is a shift we can all make. When we eat antioxidant foods, we protect our bodies from oxidative damage that shortens our lives. When we eat anti-inflammatory foods, we help our bodies heal from the daily activities and stresses that are an inevitable and important part of life (no stress = no challenge = boring life). The other hormetic tactics I share here are equally powerful in their capacity to help us heal and spark our wellbeing. Heat and cold are wonderful in small doses, as is sunlight. Gratitude practice is healing for our minds and souls.

This chapter has been all about cultivating practices in your life that give you energy, so that you can direct that energy to what matters to you the most. Recently, for me, that has been healing. As I enter the next decade of my life, I imagine that will remain my focus. I want to have the energy needed to be healthy, to make an impact in the world, and to be the best father, husband, and friend I can be to those I love.

I know the practices I shared in this chapter will help you do the same.

STANDING ON THE SHOULDERS OF GIANTS

Dr. Robyne Hanley-Dafoe on Psychological Fatigue

Dr. Robyne Hanley-Dafoe is a mental health and resiliency expert. She is a multi-award-winning psychology and education instructor who specializes in navigating stress and change, leadership, and personal wellness. I was fortunate to be able to sit down with Dr. Hanley-Dafoe on my podcast. Here is an excerpt of the conversation, in which we discuss dealing with psychological fatigue and how to use active recovery as a tool when our resources are depleted and we're reacting instead of responding.

What we start to see is we only have so much cognitive load. There's only so much we can think about, worry about, and care about. We have limits, and that doesn't mean we're not strong, capable people or resilient people. We need to know that there is an outer fray of our emotional, mental, and spiritual health. There are limits to what we can handle.

What I encourage people to think about is to use some of those micro-moments of reacting or lashing out as data. Instead of holding shame or guilt, practise some self-compassion and say, "Okay, you know what? That's data. That tells me I am running on empty, and I'm depleted. I need to do some active recovery."

I hear people say, "Oh my gosh, I need a break. Robyne, I'm done. I'm spent." We must do the work to make sure we don't get there. If you want to achieve and maintain excellence, you have to be the captain of that. No EAP program, no corporate structure, is going to solve all of this for anyone. The people who are building in active recovery, who are thinking about systems for self-repair, those are the folks who are navigating this quite readily.

To learn more, check out Dr. Robyne's incredible book Calm Within the Storm.

THRIVE

CRAFTING YOUR LIFE OF HEALTH, WELLBEING, AND PERFORMANCE

*My mission in life is not merely to survive, but to thrive;
and to do so with some passion, some compassion,
some humor, and some style.*
—MAYA ANGELOU

In highly stressful situations, or even under the pressures of daily life, some of us crumble or merely survive while others thrive. Whether these pressures are occupational, familial, financial, social, or health related, they can have damaging consequences on our overall health and wellbeing. One such consequence I've been focusing on throughout this book is burnout, which has become increasingly prevalent in recent years. In fact, according to the Global Workplace Burnout Study, 35% of respondents, representing 30 different countries, reported experiencing burnout in 2021, up from 30% in 2020.[1] Among those who reported burnout, overall wellbeing was rated at 31 out of 100, compared with a rate of 66 out of 100 in participants who did not experience burnout. With global trends of burnout on the rise, it has become more important than ever to address this crisis and find a way to thrive.

So what does it mean to thrive? And how do we achieve this state?

Let's start with a conceptual definition of thriving and what it entails. Over the past few decades, many researchers have worked to pinpoint thriving, and two common themes have emerged: development and success.[2] Development refers to progression in physical abilities (e.g., learning to play a sport), psychological abilities (e.g., learning coping strategies), and social abilities (e.g., making new friends), while success refers to achievements and positive outcomes (e.g., health, test scores, wealth). Both development and success can be predicted by high levels of emotional, psychological, or social wellbeing, as well as performance on academic, occupational, artistic, athletic, and cognitive tasks, among others.[3]

You can thrive in a specific area of your life or globally, across all areas, and thriving can occur in the pursuit of greater opportunities for growth and development.[4] It is also not dependent on overcoming adversity, which is what distinguishes thriving from concepts like resilience or stress-related growth, both of which can lead to wellbeing and success.[5] Thriving also differs from the closely related concept of flourishing because it encapsulates not only psychosocial or emotional wellbeing but also physical and mental wellbeing, as well as a performance aspect.[6] Thriving can therefore be defined as "the joint experience of development and success."

How do we achieve development and success to enable thriving? For starters, thriving is experienced differently by everyone, and there is no simple formula that can transport you from survival mode to thriving. Instead, it must be carefully cultivated over time. Whether during adversity or times of opportunity, thriving is enabled by some combination of adopting a positive perspective, experiencing religiosity and spirituality, having a proactive personality, being motivated, seeking knowledge and learning, and developing psychological resilience and social competencies.[7]

Psychologist Dr. Ryan Niemiec describes the character strengths that form our identities and help us thrive in the face of both adversity and opportunity.[8] These strengths have strong positive effects and include cognitive reappraisal (the ability to reinterpret the meaning of an event so that it has a different emotional impact), resilience, mindfulness, and appreciation. For example, mindfulness is the result of openness, curiosity, and acceptance, all of which allow us to see not only our struggles in the current moment but also the positives as well as our personal blind spots, which allows for new possibilities to be uncovered in the future.

These strengths and traits can be cultivated to help us achieve a state of thriving. But the pathway is neither simple nor linear. That's what we'll explore throughout this chapter.

One thing is for sure: your brain health holds a critical key for your thriving. None of what takes you from surviving to thriving can happen when your brain can't get the energy it requires to meet its own demands and the demands of daily life. And I'm not talking base-level demands. I'm talking about the abundance of energy you can create if you're going to beat burnout and reach new levels of energy, performance, and wellbeing. If you're going to thrive.

That's the life you want and deserve. Let's get you there.

BREAKTHROUGH IDEA:
MITOPHAGY

By now, you're an expert in the ways your mitochondria are the "power-house of the cell" and play an important role in creating all the energy required to operate. Which of course means it is very important that they stay healthy.

Mitochondria remain healthy through a balance of new mitochondria and the removal of old and damaged mitochondria. Over time, mito-chondria will become damaged or die because of factors such as age, disease, diet, and inactivity, and these damaged or dead mitochondria must be removed for the body to function properly. How do we get rid of these dysfunctional, often dead, structures?

The process by which mitochondria are broken down and removed is called *mitophagy* and is accomplished through various cellular signal-ling mechanisms. During this process, specialized proteins within your cells detect damaged mitochondria and initiate signalling cascades. These signals recruit autophagosomes, which wrap up old cells and proteins and package them for lysozomes that destroy and digest old cells and proteins.[9]

Mitophagy is required for mitochondrial quality control and steady-state turnover, as well as to meet changing metabolic energy needs.

How Mitochondria Power Your Brain
So You Can Thrive

As you know, your brain has an incredibly high metabolic rate and is thus dependent on oxidative metabolic processes to provide energy for these demands. Mitochondrial oxidative phosphorylation produces most of this ATP, which is used by neurons for neurotransmission and plasticity processes. The mitochondria also maintain Ca^{2+} homeostasis and mediate apoptosis. Because of this, neuronal health is very sensitive to mitochondrial function, and dysfunctional mitochondria are implicated in the pathophysiology of many neurological diseases.[10]

The intricacies of synaptic transmission are heavily dependent on mitochondrial energetics. For example, in the presynaptic dendritic spine, mitochondrial oxidative phosphorylation is stimulated by Ca^{2+} uptake via the mitochondrial calcium uniporter. This process is required to power ATPases that maintain ionic membrane gradients and for the recycling of synaptic vesicles. On the postsynaptic side, the mitochondria contribute to neurotransmission by providing energetic support for protein synthesis, cytoskeletal remodelling, and AMPA receptor trafficking. These plastic processes, reliant on mitochondrial oxidative phosphorylation, facilitate learning and memory in the brain. In fact, long-term potentiation is inefficient in neurons that lack mitochondria because it is dependent on mitochondrial fission and postsynaptic Ca^{2+} uptake.

Mitochondria Ca^{2+} uptake mechanisms also regulate apoptotic processes. Excitotoxicity, a loss of neurotrophic support, and neurodegenerative diseases are some of the factors that elicit apoptosis-mediated axonal degeneration. The mitochondria integrate both pro- and anti-apoptotic signals via proteins in the B cell lymphoma 2 family, which then facilitate a programmed cell death signalling cascade that results in the activation of caspases and the subsequent destruction of cells. Mitochondrial Ca^{2+} overload also plays a role in apoptotic processes by opening the mitochondrial permeability transition pore, eliciting mitochondria swelling, causing a loss of mitochondrial membrane potential, and disrupting ATP synthesis.

Mitochondrial dysfunction is critically implicated in neurodegeneration. Indeed, various mutations in Parkinson's and Alzheimer's disease–related genes impact mitochondrial bioenergetics, dynamics, and mitostasis, eliciting maladaptive disease processes within the brain. Other degenerative conditions such as Friedreich's ataxia and hereditary spastic paraplegia, as well as cancer and aging, are also driven by mitochondrial dysfunction.[11] Furthermore, mitochondrial dysfunction can be observed in seizure-like events, with large elevations in mitochondrial Ca^{2+} concentration, a loss of mitochondrial membrane potential, and increased ROS production contributing to seizure-induced cell loss. In this way, the mitochondria are critical mediators of neuronal and overall brain health.

Neurodegenerative diseases (NDs) are a group of diseases in which there is a progressive decline in nervous system function over time, such as Alzheimer's disease, Parkinson's disease, Huntington's disease, and amyotrophic lateral sclerosis. Whether mitochondrial dysfunction is a cause or consequence of these diseases is debated; however, its involvement in the pathophysiology of NDs is clear.[12,13] Aging is the greatest risk factor for developing a neurodegenerative disease, and mitochondrial dysfunction contributes to aging, through the accumulation of mitochondrial DNA (mtDNA) mutations and oxidative stress.[14]

Many neurodegenerative diseases are characterized by the accumulation of toxic proteins that cause damage to nerve cells, including the most common NDs, Alzheimer's disease and Parkinson's disease.[15] Alzheimer's disease is the most prevalent neurogenerative disease and most common type of dementia. It is characterized by a gradual loss of nerve cells in the brain, leading to a loss in memory. It is hypothesized that abnormal protein folding leads to the accumulation of amyloid plaques and tau proteins that disrupt mitochondria function, leading to an increase in ROS, cellular damage, and mtDNA mutations.[16] It is also hypothesized that the accumulation of proteins affects the mitochondrial quality control process. Impaired mitophagy prevents defective mitochondria from being removed from the cell, leading to the accumulation of defective mitochondria, further accumulation of proteins, and eventual cell death.

Parkinson's disease is characterized by muscle stiffness and rigidity, owing to the loss of dopamine-releasing neurons in the brain. It is associated with an accumulation of the protein alpha-synuclein, which is thought to damage mitochondria, leading to oxidative stress that damages nerve cells.[17] Impaired mitochondrial quality control is also suggested to be involved in this disease, and mutations in two genes that control mitophagy have been found in individuals with early-onset Parkinson's.[18]

The brain is very metabolically active and relies almost exclusively on oxidative metabolism for its energy. This also makes it particularly susceptible to oxidative stress and mitochondrial damage. Whether it is the cause or consequence of dysfunctional mitochondria, accumulation of toxic proteins, as seen in Alzheimer's and Parkinson's disease, damages mitochondria further, increases the production of ROS, and creates a feed-forward cycle of oxidative stress, cell death, and gradual loss of nervous system function.

The Challenge: Languishing

Since the beginning of the global COVID-19 pandemic, there has been a resurgence of research into various aspects of mental health, especially with respect to the positive psychological concepts of "languishing" and "flourishing."[19] Described as the "dominant emotion" in the most-read *New York Times* article of 2021,[20] languishing describes a state of being in which you feel worthless, despondent, drained, and stagnant. These are feelings that most of us can certainly identify with.

The concept of languishing was first popularized in an influential paper published in 2002 by sociologist Corey Keyes, who defined it as the absence of mental health.[21] Keyes' languishing exists on the continuum between depression and flourishing and is experienced as a lack of motivation, the inability to function properly, and a general absence of wellbeing. Keyes found that languishing was associated with impairments in psychosocial functioning, including perceived mental health, work, and other activities of daily living. These impairments were at the same level as those seen in people with depression but without any apparent or diagnosable mental illness. So those experiencing languishing did not have genuine mental health and occupied some middle ground on the mental health to illness spectrum.

Although not exactly the same as depression, anxiety, or other mental health illnesses, multiple studies have shown that languishing is closely related to these conditions and leaves people vulnerable to mental illness down the road. For example, in a study conducted in 2010, Keyes and colleagues found that languishing predicted major depressive disorder, generalized anxiety disorder, and panic disorder later in life.[22] Similarly, a 2021 study of Italian health care workers during the beginning of the pandemic found that those in a state of languishing were three times more likely to develop post-traumatic stress disorder, while flourishing emerged as a protective factor.[23]

There seem to be many risk factors for languishing. For example, one study demonstrated that first-year university students were more vulnerable to languishing, which was linked to social isolation, facing the unknown, and challenging academics, among other causes.[24] Likewise, an international study in 2020 on the effects of COVID-19 found that 10% of the study population were languishing during the first period of lockdown, associated with stresses related to social support, family functioning, and psychological flexibility.[25] Yet another study reported that languishing, or a loss of positive mental health over 10 years, was associated with lower odds of recovery from mental illness than were either moderate or positive mental health.[26] All these studies illustrate a need for public health interventions or social programs to encourage psychological, social, and emotional wellbeing among at-risk populations.

Along with the pandemic came a renewed interest in exploring potential antidotes for languishing. Some of these strategies include achieving flow state, eliminating distractions, setting goals, and exercising. The prevalence of languishing, which is the absence of mental health, is greater than that of major depressive disorder. It has now become a silent epidemic, demonstrating the need for accessible strategies to promote mental wellbeing.

STANDING ON THE SHOULDERS OF GIANTS

Dr. Milena Braticevic on Non-dual Awareness for Mental Health

Dr. Milena Braticevic has a Ph.D. in integral health from the California Institute for Human Science. She focuses on prevention-oriented methodologies for mental health sustainability and wellbeing. Her research on the effects of increasing awareness of non-dual consciousness and the natural state in young adults showed significant reductions in symptoms of depression and anxiety and increases in critical thinking, creativity, and collaboration. She currently teaches her experiential mental resilience program at corporations and educational institutions, including the University of Toronto School of Continuing Studies.

With non-duality, we can go beyond the thinking mind to experience reality more directly.

You need to be connected, so non-duality is the ultimate factor. We are so interconnected that we just think we are separate, but we are completely interconnected.

That's why when you are in a non-dual paradigm the question is no longer "How will something affect me?" but "How will I relate to everything that's happening around me?" and "How is it affecting everyone, and how are we going to collaborate to resolve a crisis?"

Maybe one of the most important things is that we need to learn to access that natural part of ourselves that's relaxed, that's authentic, where we feel that we have a sense of who we are, a healthy sense of self in connection with everyone else, then we can go from there.

A lot of times, practising that non-dual muscle means letting go of that chatter in the mind and going into more of a sense of being as opposed to doing all the time, because we are so conditioned to just achieve, and be successful, and do, and be on the go all the time.

That's not sustainable energetically, so it's very important to practise that relaxation muscle in getting to that natural state, and then when we have something to do we can be effective and we can do it with purpose and with energy.

Listen to the complete interview on my podcast at https://bit.ly /DrBraticevic.

The Opportunity: Flourishing and Thriving

You must find the place inside yourself where nothing is impossible.
—Deepak Chopra

Flourishing can be thought of as optimal mental health or the absence of mental illness, involving high levels of wellbeing, positive emotion, and optimal psychological and social functioning. In positive psychology terms, flourishing and thriving are the opposite of languishing and are embodied by a sense of purpose, fulfillment, and happiness in all aspects of life.[27] According to researchers Barbara Fredrickson and Marcial Losada, to thrive "connotates goodness, generativity, growth, and resilience."[28] As such, flourishing and thriving are an attractive state of being, though difficult to achieve, especially when stuck in a languishing rut. In fact, in a 2002 study, Keyes found that as little as 17% of the American population was flourishing, demonstrating the need for effective mental health interventions and practices that encourage wellbeing among individuals in all walks of life.[29]

The literature surrounding thriving and wellbeing is extensive, especially with the rising prevalence of the global burden of mental health illnesses. Predictors of thriving and flourishing range from personality or biological traits to demographic and socio-economic factors, and there is no "one size fits all" model to predict wellbeing.[30] For example, one study found that hopelessness mediated the relationship between social connectedness and flourishing, and individuals who were poorly connected were more likely to feel hopelessness, thus decreasing their chance of achieving a state of thriving.[31] A 2022 study found that high levels of psychological capital—a state made up of hope, efficacy, resilience, and optimism—predicted the association between organizational support and flourishing in the workplace.[32] It is therefore important to consider the multifaceted nature of mental health and wellbeing through a biopsychosocial lens to understand what enables these states of health and illness.

Current mental-health-care practices focus mainly on interventions for those people with either a diagnosable mental health disorder or identified as high risk. Such a narrow focus on mental health care illustrates the need for practical and effective everyday interventions that allow all of us to move from a state of languishing to flourishing and thriving. Several approaches have been suggested, including mindfulness, gratitude, finding purpose, getting into a state of flow, and connecting with others. However, exercise may be an even more simple option.[33]

Research shows there is a bidirectional relationship between exercise and wellbeing. For example, a longitudinal population-based study of American adults found that having a higher sense of purpose was associated with increased levels of physical activity, and that physical activity levels were positively associated with purpose four years later and also at a nine-year follow-up.[34] A similar relationship was found between exercise and mental health in a population of Seventh-Day Adventists.[35] As we've explored in other chapters, exercise continues to show up in the research as a way to improve not only your physical health but your mental health and wellbeing too.

The takeaway from all this research? Stay positive, find ways to connect with others, and exercise your mind and your body, and you will be that many steps closer to flourishing. Let's explore some specific ways in which we can move from languishing to thriving.

Thrive Practices

*I love those who can smile in trouble, who can gather strength ·
from distress, and grow brave by reflection. 'Tis the business of little
minds to shrink, but they whose heart is firm, and whose conscience
approves their conduct, will pursue their principles unto death.*
—Leonardo da Vinci

However we consider the relationship between thriving and flourishing, there is much they have in common, including, in my opinion, the most important overlap, which is that they are positive states of being that can be deliberately cultivated. What I mean is that we can actively pursue a state of thriving. We can put in place the conditions, as best as possible, to ascend from surviving to thriving.

Remember the two main conditions of thriving: development and success. Development is about moving step by step toward a more advanced state, such as fostering greater understanding or awareness of something. Success is about earning achievements that produce a positive outcome, such as becoming better at playing the piano.

Thrive practices touch on both these areas. They illustrate ways we can broaden or deepen our perspective, expand our spirituality, be proactive in our life choices, find internal motivation to change and grow, acquire greater knowledge and learning, develop resilience, and connect better to others. That's the basic development list. They also put us into the right contexts to achieve more in our lives: environments that challenge us and relationships based on attachment, trust, and support. That's the success part of the equation.

Remember mitophagy? There is a logical connection between that cellular process and the human ability to thrive that I'm describing here. Mitophagy is the process whereby old and damaged mitochondria are broken down and removed so your brain and body can function properly and maintain health. It's an ongoing process you can influence through proper rest, moving your body, eating well, taking care of your spiritual and emotional needs, and so on—all of the positive practices we've been exploring throughout this book. You can build your mitochondrial health. In response, your mitochondrial health can help build a life of thriving.

You can also think of mitophagy as a metaphor for change. As with damaged cells, we can intentionally break down and remove bad habits by replacing them, one by one, with good habits that build our health. That's what thrive practices are for. They replace old and busted systems that take away from our wellness with new and better ones that contribute to our wellness.

POWER-UP #1: CONNECT DEEPLY (COMMUNITY AND COMMUNICATION)

Isolation and lack of social connection during the COVID-19 pandemic has taken a huge toll on everyone's mental health.[36] However, loneliness was a problem well before the pandemic. This "loneliness epidemic" is such a widespread issue that the World Health Organization has raised it as one of the greatest health concerns of our time. In fact, loneliness is an independent risk factor for all-cause mortality and has been linked to morbidities such as cardiovascular disease, type 2 diabetes, depression and anxiety, suicidality and addiction, and cognitive impairments.[37]

Humans have evolved as social creatures. Connectedness (or the need to belong or have close relationships) is suggested to be one of our basic human needs—along with autonomy (the need for agency or taking control of one's life) and competence (having the proper skills and resources).[38] By engaging in social behaviour, we release oxytocin, the "bonding hormone," and other hormones associated with positive emotions and mood regulation. Indeed, many studies have highlighted the power of social connection on mental health. A study in the UK looking at over 4,000 men found that being part of a group (organization, club, society, etc.) can significantly decrease the risk of developing depression and can also improve symptoms in those already diagnosed with depression.[39] Being part of a group has been shown to reduce symptoms of post-traumatic stress, and aging adults with social support are better able to take care of themselves.[40]

Social connection has also been shown to improve physical health. A study on individuals with type 2 diabetes found that people who joined a six-month social connection intervention had significantly lower blood glucose compared with the control group.[41] Social connection also appears to impact the longevity and quality of life in both men and women living with cancer.[42,43] In addition, in a study of 734,626 middle-aged women, researchers found that living with a partner decreased the risk of heart disease mortality compared with living alone.[44] The power of social connectedness is so profound that some research indicates it might be even more important than other lifestyle factors such as smoking, alcohol consumption, physical activity, and obesity on mortality risk.[45]

This improved health and longevity can at least partly be explained by the relationship between social connectedness and the immune system. A study found that students who were lonely had a lower immune response after receiving a flu vaccine compared with those students with a strong social network.[46] So having strong social ties boosts your immune system, allowing you to fight off diseases and infections.

There is extensive evidence that social connection improves both physical and mental health outcomes. Given the toll that isolation has had on our mental wellbeing over the past few years, the need to develop social connections is apparent now more than ever. Here are some guidelines to help you.

START HERE: GET ORGANIZED

I'm sure you've heard the expression that failing to plan is planning to fail. If connecting deeply with others is going to get some priority in your life, you'll need to treat it as you do other priorities, starting with making time.

Schedule socializing into your day. In a paper published in the

American Journal of Lifestyle Medicine, the authors argue that human connection is a vital human need. They say that medical professionals should be prescribing "social connection" in the same way that exercise is prescribed and suggest using the FITT principle:[47]

Frequency: How often should social interaction occur? (e.g., daily, weekly, monthly)

Intensity: What is the quality of the social interaction? (e.g., is it a new connection, is it a shared activity, is there a deep connection)

Time: How long is the social interaction? (e.g., in minutes, hours)

Type: What type of social interaction is it? (e.g., being part of a group or organization, family gathering, friend get-together, phone call)

The authors suggest that you partake in a social interaction of some kind at least once per week, but ideally daily, to reduce your risk of mortality and morbidity and significantly improve the quality of your life. Go for a walk with friends, reconnect with someone, or spend some quality time with your partner. Schedule in daily social interaction the same way you would schedule in a meeting or appointment. Put it in your calendar so you stick with it.

Quality over quantity. Increasing your social connection doesn't mean you should friend hundreds of people on social media. According to Scott Gerber, the co-author of *Superconnector: Stop Networking and Start Building Business Relationships That Matter*, it's not the number of social connections but rather the value of them that is important.[48] It's better to have a small circle of quality connections rather than many connections, because it allows you to develop stronger and more valuable relationships.

This might be a good time to take an audit of your social connections. Who gives you energy? Who supports your dreams? On the other hand, who brings you down and holds you back? One of the wonderful things we can do in our lives is choose our friend group—and even our family, since family need not be defined by blood relatives.

Be picky. Surround yourself with people who elevate you, and do the same for them.

A LITTLE MORE ADVANCED: FOCUS ON THE HOW

Hand in hand with scheduling time with the best people you know is being intentional about *how* you see them. As Marshall McLuhan famously said, the medium is the message—meaning the form of the communication you choose is part of the message itself. When it comes to connecting deeply with others, you may need to put some real effort into choosing the medium, as it has a huge impact on the quality of your relationships.

Choose face-to-face interactions more often. Even though we can connect to so many people virtually, the online world has ironically caused more loneliness than before.[49] One reason for this is that we relate to each other through facial recognition of emotion. We can't get the same quality of connection with someone over social media or email. If you can meet up with someone in person, that will create the strongest bond. If you are unable to meet up in person, doing a video chat is the next best option.

Choose the effective dose of technology. We have never been more connected via technology, yet at the same time we have never been so far apart. This strange relationship between connection on social media or our devices and loneliness is made even harder to navigate given that different people have different needs for connection and experience connection differently. Let me explain.

I think we have many levels of communication that go from simple to more complex. These levels look something like this: text messaging via SMS or direct message → voice memo via SMS or direct message → email → voice phone call → video call → live in-person meeting.

In business situations, I recommend using the minimum effective dose of technology. Simply put, as little communication as needed in a format that is as fast as possible. Jim Donald, the former CEO of Starbucks, told me about how he communicated with everyone working at Starbucks all over the world. Each morning, he would record a 40- to 50-second voice memo about his thoughts for the day and SMS it to over 25,000 people. Simple, relatable, and effective.

The factor to consider is the relationship status of the person you are communicating with. If you are building a relationship, then you will need to have more direct contact for greater amounts of time to build trust and understanding. For established strong relationships, shorter and faster messages will work.

The caveat to all of this, especially as it relates to a post-pandemic world, is that we have learned that introverts and extroverts like to communicate differently. Further, the method of communication has opposite effects on them.

Consider the communications ladder. For an extrovert, the desired and energizing order might look like this:

SMS → DM → voice memo → voice call → video call → in-person meeting
LOW ENERGY   HIGHLY ENERGIZING

For an introvert, the ladder is reversed:

In-person meeting → video call → voice call → voice memo → DM → SMS
LOW ENERGY   HIGHLY ENERGIZING

This is why some people were thrilled to get back to working in an office after the COVID-19 pandemic and other people were devastated to have to work anywhere but at home where they could be alone and safe.

My wife and I are perfect examples of how people experience this differently. I am more of an introvert than I realized and enjoy getting most of my work done from my studio at home (although I do love presenting live and in person to thousands of people on stages all over the world). Judith loves her job as a chiropractor because she can see people live and in person and have conversations about health and wellbeing with her patients. Having face-to-face meetings all day long would be exhausting for me, but it is energizing for Judith.

Take the time to grow your awareness of what helps you thrive and how others whom you live and work with may have a different experience. We are all humans, so we can adjust and adapt the best we can. But with greater awareness, you can be intentional, effective, and healthy at the same time.

Make seeing people live your first priority, and then be selective about what technology you use to connect to others. You may need to "retrain" some people in your life when it comes to tech use, but if they're the right people for you, they will gladly come along on your journey—or at least meet you halfway.

POWER-UP #2: MAKE ROOM FOR MINDFULNESS (UNPLUG AND DISCONNECT)

Do you feel stressed to be away from your phone, or feel a need to check it all the time? Are you waiting for the notifications to pop up? You aren't the only one. It is not unusual to feel anxious and stressed when away from your phone. The *Wall Street Journal* revealed that those who run social media (Snapchat, Facebook, Instagram, Twitter, TikTok) are aware that their platforms are "toxic" for teenagers.[50]

Social media has been designed to provide immediate pleasure and reduce negative feelings; it has the same effects as alcohol or eating your favourite food.[51] In fact, social media targets the same part of your brain as addiction. The addiction pathway in the brain includes the "feel better" pathway that reinforces the experience you are having, the "must do" pathway that makes your behaviour compulsive, and the "stop now" pathway that allows you to use self-control and stop; people with addiction have an imbalance between the driving paths and self-control.[52] For example, at first you will experience a desire to use your phone because it produces feelings of happiness and entertainment. These feelings reinforce the behaviour so it becomes compulsive, and you then feel the need to be on your phone all the time. Then you lose self-control and can't stop checking your phone.

There are several reasons to be cautious with screen time, social media, and video games beyond the risk of addiction.

Screen time can negatively impact your brain function and development. Increased screen time is associated with poorer language development, memory, and attention span, which may be the result of decreased brain connectivity and decreased white matter.[53] Screen time and video games also have negative effects on emotional and social intelligence. Individuals who play violent video games have shown a delayed ability to recognize facial expressions, especially happiness. Spending more time with digital media limits face-to-face communication, which may explain why individuals with increased screen time show disrupted social and emotional intelligence.

Finally, digital media use also disrupts sleep. In both children and adolescents, increased phone use and screen time was associated with greater sleep disturbances and altered sleep onset, duration, and nighttime awakening.[54] This is a concern because poor sleep quality is associated with reduced functional connectivity and grey matter volume, which increases the risk of age-related brain impairment and disease. So next time you think about scrolling through social media or turning on your console to play a video game, hang out with a friend instead. Your brain will thank you.

You may feel discouraged about the negative effects of screen time. However, it doesn't mean you need to throw away your phone to feel better. The internet has many benefits too. Text reading and educational and active learning apps can help activate brain regions that control language, reading, and memory, and it can strengthen neural circuits. For example, searching the internet may act as a brain exercise that will increase white matter integrity to improve your brain power. Research has also shown that internet searches can increase reaction times by activating the middle frontal cortex.[55]

You may have also noticed that mental health support and interventions are now more readily accessible through technology. Technology has provided a platform that is cost-effective for mental health services and provides interventions and skills to help people manage their mental health. For example, using a cognitive behavioural therapy web-based intervention along with the usual depression care significantly improved depressive symptoms. So if you are feeling down, anxious, or stressed, try downloading a new mental health app and build lifelong skills.

We know that technology has changed the way the world works. The internet, smart phones, emails, and wearable devices put information right at our fingertips. We can have almost any product or service instantaneously. We can also stay connected to each other in a way that wasn't possible before—and, as discussed, that's not always a bonus. More connection doesn't necessarily mean better-quality connection.

And there are other downsides. Having your phone constantly by your side means you are always reachable, always available, always "on." As suggested already, social media and internet use can lead to the same destructive neural pathways as drug addictions. And having easy access to so much information means we aren't retaining knowledge in the same way we used to. This overload of technology, information, and screen time has led to three major problems: distraction, addiction, and long-term cognitive impairments. I've already touched on all of these.

It almost goes without saying that all this technology interferes with maintaining mindfulness. Remember, mindfulness means being fully present to the moment and to the self. We are aware of our thoughts, feelings, bodily sensations, and environment through a lens of calm acceptance. Being immersed in technology is pretty much the antithesis of mindfulness—it literally distracts us from that healthy awareness that keeps us from feeling overwhelmed.

So let's focus on what we can do to thrive through a balanced relationship with technology. In your life, I'm guessing that doesn't mean adding more technology time. Instead, my suggestion is to add some time to unplug and disconnect—so you can reconnect to your inner life.

START HERE: SMALL ACTS OF DISCONNECTION

In the book *The Power of Habit: Why We Do What We Do in Life and Business*, Charles Duhigg explains that 40% to 45% of the "decisions" we make every day are not actually choices—they are automatic behaviours.[56] We fall into these automatic behaviours or habits because we are programmed to conserve energy. We can't sustain a heightened level of mental focus and attention all the time.

However, once we start to recognize bad habits, we can start to make a change. The first step is to notice when you fall into destructive cycles so you can plan to avoid them and start replacing them with more mindful habits. It takes time and discipline, but small changes really do pay off. Here are some suggestions for getting started.

Make sure all phones are put away at family dinners. This also means making sure your notifications are turned off, so you don't hear your phone going off. You should disable notifications on any wearable devices as well.

Turn off phone and email notifications when doing important work. One of the main sources of distractions for employees is getting emails and texts throughout the day. During work, especially when you need to really focus, put away your phone and turn off notifications on both your computer and phone.

Batch your emails. Instead of constantly checking and replying to emails while you're trying to get work done, set aside specific times of the day to check and respond to emails. For some of you, we realize that emails are a bigger part of your work, and you might need to check them more regularly. However, for most of us, checking emails every 20 minutes is not necessary and incredibly inefficient. Instead, dedicate two or three times per day to emails and dedicate the other parts of your day to important work.

Build media time into your schedule. Build screen time into your day to give yourself a sense of control and to set realistic expectations. For example, maybe you allow yourself to watch a show after dinner or dedicate specific times of the day to going on social media. You might want to set a timer and, once it goes off, it's time to get back to whatever is next in your daily schedule.

Make an #unplug challenge with friends. When spending time with your friends or family, challenge everyone to put their devices away for a chunk of time—maybe while at the park or while having people over for your famous Bolognese . . . Just an hour or two of absolutely no one looking at their devices can be incredibly mentally and emotionally refreshing.

A LITTLE MORE ADVANCED: DISCONNECT MORE DEEPLY

Let's take this concept to another level by building practices into our lives that help us to disconnect, reconnect, and recharge more deeply more often.

Don't bring your phone into your bedroom. Researchers have found that children who used media devices before bed had an increased likelihood of inadequate sleep, poor sleep quality, and excessive daytime sleepiness.[57] Even having the device in the room was associated with detrimental sleep effects, which is why it's important to not even bring your phone into the bedroom. Invest in an alarm clock and use that to wake yourself up instead.

Take a full day to unplug. If you're like me, you're probably regularly bombarded with phone calls, messages, and news. It's important to step away from all that and be fully unplugged for good stretches of time. If you're going through a period of high stress, leave your phone at home and go for a walk or even a day-long hike and just enjoy being disconnected. You may need to plan ahead to take a full day off from your phone, but it's worth it. This dose of device-free time will ease some of your psychological stress, reconnect you to yourself and your real-world surroundings, and leave you feeling refreshed.

Take a real vacation. A vacation isn't *really* a vacation if we never completely disconnect from work life or other habitual tech uses. Unfortunately, it has become the norm for many of us to stay connected to work, and just the idea of vacation sends some of us into a panic. Since the thought of being "disconnected" makes most people anxious, they either don't go away at all or they take their work with them. But as you know, this is detrimental to your mental health, and it also hurts productivity in the long run.

Here are three ideas for you that can help make a real vacation a reality:

1. Make sure your work will be taken care of while you are away.
Let your team, co-workers, and boss know that you are going away and won't be able to check your devices.

2. Use your "out of office" email. Turn on the vacation notice in your email, including a note that says something like "I am currently on vacation. I will not be checking my email while I am away from the office. If you need immediate assistance please contact my colleague, who will be able to assist you." Then give yourself permission to not check your messages while you are away.

3. Consciously disconnect. This goes beyond work to all your technology habits. Most of us don't ever make a conscious decision to entirely disconnect (though maybe you've taken me up on the challenge and have tried a full day). Make a promise to yourself to get unstuck from a perpetual state of device slavery that has become habitual, compulsive, and, ultimately, a drain on your resources and relationships. Use your vacation as an excuse to disconnect and to be completely unplugged (for both work and personal purposes).

STANDING ON THE SHOULDERS OF GIANTS

Tia Slightham on Avoiding Screen-Time Battles with Your Kids

Tia Slightham works with parents to teach positive ways to decrease the daily struggles we all encounter as parents. Tia has a master's degree in early childhood education, is certified in positive discipline, and has worked with kids and families for over 17 years. Here are her tips for stopping screen-time battles with your kids:

Open communication. It's important to chat with your kids up front about the pros and cons of technology. The more open you are with your kids the better. If your kids refuse to discuss this with you, then you will need to open the door to communication by starting slow. Ask one question from time to time.

Set respectful limitations in advance. Limitations need to be age appropriate. If you have a toddler or young child who is always wanting to use your phone, TV, or iPad, then it's important to set boundaries and limitations in advance. Communicate with them your concerns about technology and let them know limits are not being set to be "mean" but rather are in their best interest. They may not agree, but you are the parent and do know best. When setting limits, it's extremely important to be fair. For example, "Once your homework is done each day, you can watch the television."

Offer choice. Give your kids choice around when they can use technology. For example, "Do you want to watch your show after school or before bed?" Giving choice will take away some of the pushback. It will give your kids a chance to have some power and control over their own world.

Follow through. If you set a boundary in advance, you must follow through. Consequences that are fair will be highly effective if you follow through.

Model what you teach. Do what you want your kids to do. If you want to respect your kids and your kids to respect you, then you must be fair. If phones are not allowed at the table, then you must not be checking your device either. If technology is a problem in your home, then the first step to fixing this issue is *you*.

You can learn more and connect directly with Tia at www.tiaslightham.com.

POWER-UP #3: HAVE FUN

Happiness and health are highly correlated. Happy people tend to be healthier physically and have a lower risk of developing chronic diseases.[58] A study on individuals with type 2 diabetes found that those who were happier had lower inflammatory markers, which might slow the progression of the disease.[59] Happy people have also been shown to be more productive at work,[60] and there is even some research suggesting that happiness can improve mitochondrial health.[61]

Research on twins suggests that 35% to 50% of happiness is genetic.[62] This means that while a lot of our happiness is out of our control, there is still a lot that is in our control. The catch is that, according to a conversation I had with Dr. Gillian Mandich, who studies the science of happiness, humans aren't great at knowing what makes them happy. She says it's not the big shiny moments, such as a promotion or new car, but rather the small moments that add up over time that determine how happy we are.

Dr. Michael Rucker, another expert in the field of happiness I had the pleasure of chatting with, says that the Goldilocks spot is to dedicate at least two hours per day (14 hours per week) to pleasurable activities. This might mean carving out some time for a specific fun activity or learning how to find pleasure in an activity you're already doing.

Like many other things, happiness is a learned skill that we must practise. But eventually it will become habit and you'll be in a positive state more often.

So how can we invite more happiness into our lives?

START HERE: SMALL OUTBREAKS OF FUN

Keep in mind how powerful it can be to make small changes to less-than-ideal habits.

Sprinkle in small bursts of joy. The sum of small day-to-day moments create a happy life. So one way to invite more happiness into your life is to sprinkle in small bursts of joy throughout the day. This might mean emailing someone to thank them for something they did for you, having a meaningful conversation with a friend, taking 30 seconds to help someone who needs it, or recalling a great past experience.

Seek out playful activities. Engaging in playful activities such as sports or games not only boosts your happiness but is also important for your brain. A study found that juvenile rats that engaged in "rough and tumble" play had higher activation in certain areas of the brain compared with control rats. They also had greater brain-derived neurotrophic factor (BDNF) gene expression, suggesting that play is important for neurodevelopment.[63]

Practise gratitude. I've already talked about how gratitude is about appreciating the good in your life as opposed to focusing on the negatives. It makes the list here again because, while it sounds simple, gratitude can change the way our brains are wired for the better. Practising gratitude has been shown to be associated with greater life satisfaction, improved mood, less stress, and even better athletic recovery via reducing inflammation, decreasing blood pressure, and improving sleep.[64]

Don't underestimate the power of humour. Laughing is such a powerful mood lifter that laughing therapy is being used to treat people for mental illnesses such as depression and anxiety, as well as stress-related diseases. It appears that laughter suppresses cortisol, one of the stress hormones, while enhancing dopamine and serotonin, the feel-good chemicals.[65] Give yourself some laughter therapy by going to see a stand-up comedian or an improv show, or watch your favourite comedy.

A LITTLE MORE ADVANCED:
CARVE TIME FOR SELF-CARE AND EVEN SADNESS

These suggestions take more time, planning, and even self-awareness—and provide excellent opportunities to directly or indirectly increase your overall happiness.

Make self-care non-negotiable. This means dedicating some time each day to an activity that is for you and you only. Going for that quick walk in the middle of the day will not only improve your physical health but also make you more focused the rest of the day. Taking time to meditate every day will make you more patient with your family. Setting aside time to work on a project or hobby will give you balance, give you a sense of accomplishment, and make you happier. On a larger scale, you may want to take up an activity that requires lessons or regular practice, like painting or woodworking or rock climbing. What's important is making a commitment to and then scheduling self-care activities into your life.

Don't confuse seeking happiness with trying to be happy all the time. Into every life a little rain must fall. In fact, trying to be happy all the time makes us *less* happy, because we're constantly chasing (and failing to achieve) an unrealistic expectation. Instead, focus on creating joyful moments when you can and accepting the lows as they come as well. Also, think of happiness as a result, not a pursuit in itself: it's a side effect of the choices you make about how you see and interpret events, how well you understand yourself and your needs, how much you invest in relationships and activities that fulfil you, and so on. Not only is it important to work through and embrace the learning that difficult life moments provide, it's also critical to not confuse happiness with getting everything you want. It's an outcome of perspective and effort, not a shiny bauble that can be bought and sold.

POWER-UP #4: CRAFT YOUR IKIGAI (MEANING AND PURPOSE)

Ikigai combines the Japanese words *iki*, which means "life" or "alive," and *gai*, which means "worth" or "benefit."[66] The state of ikigai is traditionally defined as that which gives your life meaning and purpose or, in other words, "what makes life worth living."[67] Ikigai is not conceptual; rather, it is experiential, and it is only experienced when you are living your mission.[68] It can also be understood through the emotional concepts of happiness and satisfaction with life and cognitive appraisal of your self-efficacy, your self-esteem, and the meaning of your life.[69] In this way, ikigai is closely related to positive psychology and may thus be cultivated through psychological intervention.

As an aging population with an above-average life expectancy, Japanese people are particularly concerned with ikigai, given that they often outlive their workplace- or family-related social roles and must therefore search for new meaning.[70] Interestingly, research shows that ikigai may have key gender differences. For example, in one study, ikigai in men was more often associated with physical condition and socio-economic factors such as income and assets, while in women it was more associated with family relations and satisfaction with life history.[71]

Principally studied within Japanese populations, ikigai has been shown to have a multitude of physical and mental health benefits.[72] To date, one of the best-studied effects of ikigai is its association with longevity. Indeed, having ikigai is associated with a decreased risk for all-cause mortality and functional and cognitive decline.[73,74,75] Other physical health benefits of ikigai include a decreased risk of disability among the elderly, improved immune functioning, better recovery following surgery, and decreased allostatic load (wear and tear on the body), among others.

Although the mechanism by which ikigai increases physical health and longevity remains uncertain, it is thought to be related to increased positive health-related behaviours and neuroendocrine, inflammatory, and immune responses. Mental health research on ikigai demonstrates it is a positive predictor of wellbeing and a negative predictor of depression. One interesting study showed that having ikigai was associated with lower sympathetic (fight or flight) nervous system activation during physiological and psychological stress and more effective coping.[76] In this way, ikigai may have therapeutic potential in chronic stress and mental health illness.[77] More research, however, is needed to elucidate the psychological and physiological effects of ikigai.

START HERE: FOLLOW THE FIVE PILLARS OF IKIGAI

Neuroscientist Ken Mogi suggests that the loss of ikigai in our lives is primarily driven by our intense fixation on external goals and rewards such as money or fame. As is thriving in general, ikigai is associated more with intrinsic motivation and quality-focused cultures rather than success-focused cultures. According to Mogi,[78] ikigai can be found in the following five pillars:

Start small. *Kodawari* is the Japanese concept of paying extraordinary care to the small details. This pillar is simple: take small steps forward and pay attention to the details, and eventually you'll achieve your goals and purpose.

Release yourself. Carefree individuals are not burdened with social definitions of the self. Releasing yourself means finding ways to be happy through acceptance of yourself, your place, and the way you engage in life.

Achieve harmony and sustainability. Achieving ikigai is rooted in being in harmony with the environment, society, and the people around you, promoting sustainability.

Find joy in the little things. The small and rewarding pleasures of life cause the release of dopamine in your brain, facilitating contentment and happiness. Forging habits of using the little things to bring us joy allows us to cultivate ikigai.

Be in the here and now. Perhaps the most profound pillar of ikigai, being in the here and now with ephemeral joy is a characteristic that ikigai shares with mindfulness. Mogi describes it as being in touch with your inner child and a creative and successful attribute that you can bring into your life and the lives of those you surround yourself with in order to cultivate ikigai.

A LITTLE MORE ADVANCED: LIFE CRAFTING

Here are other evidence-based ways to cultivate ikigai that require a little more thought and care.

Craft your life. Research shows that life crafting, an intervention based on ikigai, is associated with many physical and mental health benefits.[79] Life crafting allows you to take control of your life, find happiness, and achieve optimal performance. So what is it exactly? Life crafting includes cultivating your values and passions, becoming aware of your current and desired habits and rituals, focusing on your relationships and social life, optimizing your career path, and formulating self-concordant goals and ways to achieve them.

Stay social. Having a strong social community is a protective factor for the maintenance of ikigai as you age. Indeed, one longitudinal study showed that social capital, or the presence of strong social ties and communities, protected against declines in ikigai stemming from poor health or financial status during aging.[80]

Find flow. Flow keeps coming up because it is such a powerful concept and state of being. You know that flow happens when you are happiest and fully immersed in the task at hand, which is why it is in tune with ikigai. In a state of flow, tasks can become rewarding and can cultivate ikigai.

POWER-UP #5: CREATE A SOUNDTRACK FOR YOUR LIFE (PEAK PERFORMANCE)

If you think about how music affects us—from pumping us up to filling us with pleasure to bringing tears to our eyes—it's not hard to imagine it has a powerful effect on the brain and body. The effect of music stretches beyond the experience of sounds to influence emotions, health, and wellbeing, as well as physical and mental performance. The benefits of music can be harnessed to achieve a sense of thriving by allowing you to power up your physical and cognitive abilities.

By now, you have learned the incredible benefits of physical activity and the importance of remaining active. Listening to music while exercising has been shown to improve physical performance and decrease fatigue.[81] Fast-tempo music increases maximal power output and alters the perceptions of fatigue.[82] So next time you go on that run or head to the gym, bring your headphones.

Music has also been associated with a boost in natural killer (NK) cells and immunoglobulin A (IgA) activity, with both key components of your body's first line of defence against stress and aging.[83] Positive emotions also reduce stress and increase IgA activity to strengthen your immune system, so don't be afraid to smile while listening to your favourite music. Show your immune system some love, and support it by including music in your daily routine.

Music is also a brain booster. It has been shown to improve performance on problem solving and memory tasks and to enhance concentration.[84] Some researchers reported that children who received musical training had increased grey matter density in the right primary auditory cortex, which was associated with improved cognitive functioning.[85] Music also stimulates the brain regions involved in reward, motivation, and pleasure. Listening to "chill-inducing" and pleasurable music increases blood flow to your nucleus accumbens and ventral tegmental area in the brain, which are associated with the release of dopamine and endogenous opioids, substances that play a key role in rewarding and motivating behaviour, as well as in happiness.[86] These same brain regions are stimulated by food, sex, alcohol, and the internet.

START HERE: MUSIC FOR MENTAL PERFORMANCE

Here are some simple ways to power up your life through music.

Self-selected music. Choose your favourite song to increase your motivation, enhance your productivity, and improve your mood, since music has been found to do all three.

Fast-tempo music. Power up your workout with upbeat, fast-tempo music that will maximize your power output and reduce neuromuscular fatigue.

Drumming and relaxing music. Counteract age-related declines in immune function, while improving mood and reducing stress, with drumming and relaxing music.

Classical music. Power up your cognitive performance in school or at work by listening to classical music. Classical music improves health and wellbeing by enhancing brain activity.[87] It enhances efficiency, produces a calming and relaxing state, reduces stress, improves cell growth rates, and facilitates performance on exams and spatial puzzles.

Next time you put on your headphones, choose a playlist with some of your favourite upbeat and fast-tempo songs to power up your physical performance and positive emotions. During those relaxing times, or when concentrating at work or school, play some classical music or drumming to power up your mental performance and immune system.

A LITTLE MORE ADVANCED: SPECIFIC PLAYLISTS FOR SPECIFIC TASKS

Now you can start to build your playlists to help you accomplish specific tasks or to deliberately enhance your life during key moments. You can build a playlist for your cardio workouts, your strength workouts, or your gentle stretching sessions. We have a playlist that we put on during dinner with the family. We have another playlist that helps us all get energized in the car on the way to work and school in the morning, and a very different playlist that helps us calm down and relax at the end of the day when we are on the way home.

Think about the main areas of your life where you could benefit from the power of music. Then create your playlists to match the music to the energy you want to have in those key moments.

POWER-UP #6: PLAY (HEALTH AND WELLBEING)

Play is a ubiquitous practice across species that researchers believe evolved as a highly desired characteristic among potential mating partners.[88] For our earliest ancestors, play may have been an important way to teach adolescents the skills of cooperation and sharing that were essential for survival.[89] Today, it may serve a different purpose. Unfortunately, in many cultures, there is a prevailing notion that play is only for children. But as researchers have begun to investigate the role of play in the lives of adults, they have found it is important for health and wellbeing across all age groups.

The most important latent function of play may be stress reduction. Indeed, in a cross-sectional study of university students, playful participants reported significantly lower levels of perceived stress and demonstrated greater adaptive-oriented and fewer maladaptive-, escape-, or avoidance-oriented stress-coping strategies than their non-playful counterparts.[90] In this way, play allowed them to mobilize cognitive resources for coping in the face of stress and building resilience. Play also improves your mood, relationships, mental health, ability to cope with chronic illness, and social skills and boosts your vitality and daily levels of activity.[91] Studies show that play enhances the release of the feel-good hormones dopamine, serotonin, endorphins, and oxytocin, which work to protect mental health and wellbeing.[92]

Not only is play important for our health and wellbeing, it may also be beneficial in practical and professional settings. In the workplace, play has been shown to reduce stress and negative emotions, increase productivity and job satisfaction, and improve employee cohesion, commitment, and overall work quality.[93] For example, a 2020 study investigating a play-at-work intervention at a South African telesales company found that employees who played games such as puzzles, foosball, cards, or darts during their lunch break were better able to psychologically detach from their work than those who did not.[94] Overall team performance also increased following the intervention.

The lesson to take away from all of this? Get out and play. It not only comes with great benefits for your health, wellbeing, and career but is also fun, creative, and enjoyable. Check out these suggestions for ways to incorporate play into your life.

START HERE: BACK TO BASICS

It's time to pause and give yourself permission to have some fun. We don't need to be productive every second of every day. Relaxing and playing is powerful and just plain fun. Here are a few ideas for you to build a bit more chill and smile time back into your days.

Colour. In the last decade, adult colouring books have become a trendy new form of creative play that is beneficial for many reasons. Colouring interventions have consistently been shown to reduce negative psychological outcomes, including symptoms of depression and anxiety.[95] In fact, colouring has even been suggested as an alternative form of meditation, as it allows us to switch our brains off and relax and focus on the task at hand, which reduces any pent-up tension, stress, and anxiety.[96]

Try your hand at puzzles. Not only are puzzles a great way to wind down at the end of a long day and release built-up stress, but they also have incredible cognitive and mental health benefits. Puzzles engage your brain and have been shown to enhance memory, protect against cognitive decline and diseases such as dementia and Alzheimer's, improve problem-solving and vocabulary skills, raise IQ, and increase productivity and collaboration in a group setting.[97] Some different puzzles you can try include crosswords, jigsaw puzzles, sudoku, dominos, checkers, and chess. For an even more immersive experience, try your hand at an escape room.

Play with your pet. Have you ever heard of puppy therapy? It turns out that interacting with animals causes your body to produce the feel-good hormones serotonin and dopamine, which promote mental health and alleviate depression and anxiety. Additionally, animals can have calming and relaxing effects and encourage a healthy, playful lifestyle and all the benefits that come along with it.[98] So take some time out of your day to pet your cat, or even better, take your play outside and go for a walk or play fetch with your dog.

A LITTLE MORE ADVANCED: TRY SPORTS

You can add a little complexity by playing with others either formally (sports) or informally (just play). This helps to spark community and connection and to build a sense of team where you share common experiences with others.

Play with others. Research shows that playing with others fosters compassion, empathy, intimacy, and trust, and that play itself may have evolved as a social practice. Group play also helps us build relationships and learn to work as a team. Some great collaborative ways that you can play with others include escape rooms, board games, and organized sports.

Play outdoor games. Exercise is perhaps the most important health-promoting practice and may also be one of the reasons why play is so healthy. Living an active lifestyle where we play outside can help us feel like we are enjoying life. Just think about when you take your kids to the park, when you go for a walk in nature, or when you have a family ski day in the winter or beach day in the summer.[99] Furthermore, as mentioned earlier, being in a natural environment while you play, or getting "green exercise," imparts additional benefits such as improved mental and physiological health, a decreased risk for disease, elevated mood and self-esteem, and reduced stress, among many more.[100] Any form of green exercise is great, so on the next nice day, get out and play tennis or Frisbee, organize a soccer match, ride your bike, or fly a kite. The possibilities are endless.

POWER-UP #7: CREATE MAGIC MOMENTS

As we near the end of this book, I am thinking deeply about the ultimate objective of all my research, speaking, and writing. The foundation is elevating health and wellbeing. We can't thrive without our health. This is what I hope I have accomplished as a scientist and researcher at SickKids hospital. The next level is helping people reach their potential—to perform at their best level at what they care about the most. In my work, that has been my practice with athletes and adventurers as a performance physiologist. More recently, I am shifting my focus to making a broader difference in the world and having more of an impact on people's lives. I am shifting my efforts to help people experience more magic moments.

Magic moments are those special times when you are in a state of flow but also having an experience that is deeply meaningful for you. This is looking into the eyes of a loved one. Watching a sunset over the ocean. Walking through the woods with your kids and seeing them express wonder and awe. It can also be doing a powerful presentation that elevates your mission at work. For teachers, a magic moment might be when they help a child make a breakthrough in their understanding to have a "eureka" moment.

A leading researcher in the field of peak experience, Gayle Privette from the University of West Florida, suggests that a peak experience involves "a heightened sense of wonder, awe, or ecstasy over an experience."[101] At this point in my life, I am doing my best to create magic moments for my family. Adam loves baseball, so we go to Blue Jays games. Ingrid loves swimming, so we just got her certified as a scuba diver. Judith loves connecting with people, so we have been hosting friends at our home more often. I just love being outdoors exercising in nature, so I have been riding my mountain bike in the woods as often as possible.

Other researchers have explored this state and tried to describe peak experiences and magic life moments. Abraham Maslow, an American psychologist who is best known for creating his hierarchy of needs, described peak experiences as "powerful, meaningful experiences in which individuals seem to transcend the self, be at one with the world, and feel completely self-fulfilled." In his book *Toward a Psychology of Being*, Maslow noted that keys to peak experience include a sense of oneness, timelessness, effortlessness, playfulness, and happiness.[102]

The most important thing from my perspective in elevating a peak experience into a magic moment that is transcendent and transformative is the addition of meaning. For example, if you are on a beach watching the sun set over the ocean, that is an incredible experience. You may even drop into a state of flow. Consider the cascading effects of sharing that moment with your partner or children, then moving from flow (which is awesome) to a meaningful moment (watching your kids experience awe), which then elevates your life in that moment to a peak experience that is so magical it transcends time (you will remember that moment forever) and transforms everyone involved (your children develop a love of travel and adventure, and you know you are making a positive difference in their lives).

Everything I have shared in this book is designed to set you up for creating magic moments in your life. Breathing to settle and oxygenate your mind and body. Moving to enhance your health and wellbeing. Energizing so you are fuelled to follow your pursuits and passions. Finally, tactics for thriving in your life so you can live to your potential and have as much of a positive influence in the world as you can.

START HERE: APPRECIATE THE MOMENTS THAT ARISE

We are so busy in our lives that we often miss the magic in our rush to the next appointment or task. With full awareness of how hard life can be, I would love for you to take moments through your days, weeks, months, and years to pause—even for a few seconds—to appreciate the wonders around us.

Like . . .

- Your children learning something new
- Leaves in the trees moving and shaping the light that passes through them from the sun
- How your muscles feel as they power you up the stairs
- Reading beautifully crafted words in a book by a master
- Looking at a piece of art in your home, at a gallery, or online
- Listening to an awesome piece of music

Simply press pause on your busy life to open yourself up to the magic that exists all around us. I am writing this piece from an airport, and I just saw a couple reunite with a long hug. Magic.

A LITTLE MORE ADVANCED:
DELIBERATELY CREATE MAGIC MOMENTS

This requires a bit of intention and planning. Magic happens when we do activities we love, with people we love, and we are present in the moment. We all can benefit from more magic in our lives.

You can set up a movie night with great food and no distractions at home. You can coach your child's sports team and share words of encouragement to help them in a moment when they are experiencing pre-game nerves. You can have good friends over for a special dinner. You can play music at home. You can take your teenager for a walk and listen to them and ask questions with no agenda or judgment.

There is so much magic in the world. We can appreciate the magic as it happens to us, then create magic to share with others.

STANDING ON THE SHOULDERS OF GIANTS

Dr. Gillian Mandich on the Science of Happiness

Dr. Gillian Mandich has a Ph.D. from Western University in health science, specializing in health promotion. Her primary areas of research are happiness and health, and her work combines the latest research, practical wisdom, and engagement to help people live happier, healthier lives. Gillian is the founder of the International Happiness Institute of Health Science Research, is part of the Meant2Prevent research team at SickKids, and is the co-lead investigator of the Canadian Happiness at Work Study. In this excerpt of my podcast interview with her, Gillian discusses the dark side of happiness and how important experiencing the full palette of human emotions is for our psychological functioning.

When I first started studying happiness, I asked myself, "Gillian, are you as happy as you possibly could be?" And my answer was no . . . I don't want to feel any of these challenging emotions that I experience sometimes, I don't want to feel anxiety, I don't want to feel down or depressed. I don't want to feel sad.

I asked myself, "Why don't I study happiness and figure out how I can make myself happy?" What I quickly learned was that the goal is not to be happy all the time. That was eye-opening for me, because it allowed me to understand this palette of human emotions that are all—at certain times—healthy in terms of our psychological functioning.

In the research, it's called the dark side of happiness. Often people put on their blinders and single-mindedly, narrow-mindedly focus on happiness. Their goal is to be happy all the time. Those people are less happy than other people, which is surprising until you stop to unpack it a little bit, because if you think about it, you can't be happy all the time. That's not possible. So if that's my goal, I have set a goal that is so unrealistic and so unattainable that I will never achieve it. And so now I'm going to start feeling worse about myself because I'm now not meeting my goal, even though my goal is completely unrealistic.

So where I have gone learning all of this is recognizing that feeling emotions is the key. Whatever they are, feeling them fully, not blocking them, not ignoring them, not pushing them away. But instead, welcoming the full spectrum of human emotions.

Yes, there are times when happiness is amazing, and it can be a great time in our lives. And sometimes going through the more challenging or difficult times can test our character. It may show us a strength that we never thought was possible. There's just that mindset shift of knowing it's okay to not be happy all the time, and in fact, that's not the goal. This was so freeing for me because then I began to shift the conversation into really embracing the palette of emotions that we experience.

Listen to the complete interview on my podcast at https://bit.ly /DrGillianMandich2.

Craft a Thriving Life

The greatest glory in living lies not in never falling, but in rising every time we fall. —NELSON MANDELA

Yesterday I asked my teammate Sara Thompson at my consulting firm Wells Performance a simple but important question. I asked, "Hey, ST. If there was one thing that we do or teach— one idea that people find super helpful in our programs—what would you say that is?"

Sara answered with "I would say it's the 1% gains . . . small wins that create lasting change in the long term. All our really good testimonials are people talking about how simple ideas have helped them enormously (leaving the phone outside the bedroom, going for a daily walk, etc.). People are pleasantly surprised by how such small changes can have such a big impact."

I share this principle with you at this point in the book because the ideas I have shared here in the Thrive chapter are big ideas that can seem overwhelming. Crafting your ikigai is a process that takes time. Appreciating and creating magic moments is not something that often happens immediately or easily. These ideas are powerful and life changing, and we can instill them in our lives just a little bit at a time. That leads to exponential improvements in health and wellbeing over time.

It took me 20 years to craft the magic moment I am experiencing right now as I write these words. In 2003 I cycled across

Africa with the Tour d'Afrique cycling expedition. At the end of that trip, I imagined taking my future family (I was single, unemployed with a Ph.D., and had a load of student loans) on a safari in Tanzania. It took me 20 years to craft my ikigai, meet and marry Judith, create a family, craft a career of meaning and impact, and have fun and play with my kids to the point where we—last week—were able to travel back to Africa and have the most magical of experiences in the Serengeti plains of Tanzania. Seeing my children watch lions and cheetahs with wondrous eyes made all the ups and downs of life worth every second.

The ideas I have shared here are powerful. They can help you craft a life of health and wellbeing where you can share magical moments with those you love. These magical moments make the world a better place one little 1% step at a time.

Be consistent, stay the course, have fun, play, craft your life, and experience the magic that life offers.

THE 100-DAY
MITOCHONDRIAL CHALLENGE

A SIMPLE DAILY PLAN FOR A NEW YOU

The best way to predict the future is to create it.
—ABRAHAM LINCOLN

Your mitochondria have a lifespan of around 100 days. So in just 100 days, when you instill new, healthy practices in your life, you can expect your new mitochondria to benefit from these powerful tactics and you will have an uptick in your health, well-being, and energy.

The most successful high performers tend to use daily habits, rituals, and routines that are consistent with their dreams, goals, and objectives.

According to research by Phillippa Lally and colleagues from University College London, it takes 20 to 120 practice sessions to instill a new habit, with the average being around 66 days.[*] So for at least two months, you need to focus on instilling that one new

---

[*] "How long does it take to form a habit?" UCL News (August 4, 2009). www.ucl.ac.uk/news/2009/aug/how-long-does-it-take-form-habit.

habit until it is routine. Once you're there, you can then free up the energy required to do so and use it elsewhere.

Positive habits are routines and rituals we practise that elevate our lives. Drinking some ginger tea with lemon first thing in the morning. Going for a walk with a friend on the weekend. Writing five things you are grateful for at the end of each day in your journal. Doing yoga in the morning to loosen up your body. When the positive habit is practised consistently, it becomes a routine. When your routines are matched to what is meaningful for you in your life (e.g., morning yoga matched to your desire to get healthy), it becomes a ritual. Positive habits, routines, and rituals all protect our energy, optimize our mental and physical health, and enable us to perform to our potential consistently and sustainably.

Start with small habits. After injuries, athletes get right back to the basics and rebuild their health, fitness, and performance from the ground up. You can do exactly the same thing. Go for a 15-minute walk. Do some simple exercises. Take a yoga class. Just get active. Start very small and build from there. Micro-wins win.

Be consistent and you will craft powerful routines. Olympians build their strength, flexibility, balance, and cardiorespiratory fitness over thousands of hours and many years of deliberate practice and training. So don't worry about it if you get off track for a while. The key is to get back to being active as soon as you can. When you start again, you might get frustrated. But each time you get going, your health, wellbeing, and performance will come back faster and faster.

Build your supercharging rituals. Make your positive activities part of your routine. Book time in your calendar. Make them a priority. Shift away from your busy to-do list and direct your attention and time to your priorities. That way you won't have to decide whether to do them when you're busy or if you get tired during your day.

Remember that a little is good and a lot is not. Counterintuitively, life optimization isn't about big, dramatic changes. You can't leap 10 miles at a time. You can't move ahead to next week or next month or next year. All you can do is give this moment—this day—your full attention and intention. When you do that, it is easy to apply your attention to your vision and dreams so that you can build revolutionary rituals.

I've chosen simple things you can do each day. Just follow along and do your best. If you miss a day, no worries at all, just start up where you left off. Even if this takes a year, it will still help you. So stick with this for 100 days and you will have your new mitochondria-friendly lifestyle to power you into a new future.

As you move along your journey you can share your progress with me on Twitter or Instagram @drgregwells. You can also message me via my website at www.drgregwells.com. I can't wait to follow you on your journey.

If you want me to send you a note each morning for 100 days to remind you of what the challenge of the day is, you can sign up at www.drgregwells.com/100daymitochallenge.

You can track your sleep, movement, nutrition, and recharging using our free VIIVIO app (download at www.viiv.io).

Day 1. Set Your Intentions

When we have clarity about our intentions and direction in our lives, we can make the right decisions at the right time to ensure that our actions are consistent with our intentions.

So what are your intentions for the next 100 days? Here are some examples:

"I will take five minutes each day for myself."

"I will complete this 100-day challenge."

"I will put myself first so I can be my best for those I love."

Be specific. What *will* you do?

Write your intentions on a coloured sticky note and post it somewhere at home, in your car, or at the office (or all three) where you will see it every day.

Completed! [   ]

Day 2. Take Three Deep Breaths

Place a hand on your belly and inhale deeply, filling your belly with your breath. Pause. Then exhale slowly to the count of seven. Try that once more, making sure your exhale is gentle and slow. Repeat one more time.

You just practised mindful breathing and, in the process, calmed down your nervous system. Moving forward, use these three deep breaths to bring yourself a sense of calm when you are stressed or anxious. It's easy to do this when you are rested and chill. It is more challenging to do when you are having a difficult moment. But it is in these moments of challenge where the true power of this technique will reveal itself.

Completed! [   ]

Day 3. Go for a Walk

Take a short walk outside (even five minutes is fantastic). Please keep it short. Do less than you think you need to and less than you want to. Leave yourself wanting more.

I'm looking for you to begin creating the habit of directing energy and time toward you. Your health. Your wellbeing. So taking 5 to 10 minutes to go for a walk, even though it seems like a microtask, can spark a radical long-term shift.

Here is where it gets hard—leave your phone at home so you can be totally present in your walk and able to focus on what's around you. You will be fine. And if something goes wrong, everyone else around you will have a phone.

Completed! [   ]

Day 4. Take a Hot Bath

It's time to leverage that heat is a powerful stimulus for positive adaptation in the human body. So take a hot bath and relax.

Give yourself 10 to 20 minutes. Fill the tub with hot water and get it to the point where you notice it is as hot as you can handle while still being relaxing and comfortable. Get the bubbles going. Light a candle. Burn some incense. Play some chill music. PS: If you don't have a bathtub, no worries, just take a long hot shower.

Give yourself a break. Heat your body up. Spark your mitochondria.

Completed! [   ]

Day 5. Avengers Assemble

I love Marvel movies. There is a moment in an Avengers movie where Captain America says the classic line from the comics: "Avengers . . . assemble." This is when the team of superheroes have all come together. Captain America, Spider-Man, the Incredible Hulk, they are all there. And they save the world.

Who are the people in your life that are powerful positive influences on you? Who in your circle elevates each other?

If you don't have any close friends right now who are positive influences, that's totally okay. Who can you follow online that truly elevates you in a positive way? What podcast can you listen to that is constructive, positive, and informative and that, when you listen to the show, helps you be better?

Now that you have an idea of the people who are positive influences in your life, let's start to assemble those people. Call your friend. Send a quick SMS. Just say hello. Subscribe to the podcast. DM the podcast show host on social and let them know that you are listening and that you enjoy the show.

Reach out with no expectation. We are simply beginning to assemble our own superhero team.

Completed! [   ]

Day 6. Practise 2:4:6 Breathing

First, find a special place where you can sit comfortably, or lie down (on a yoga mat if you'd like).

Bring your attention to your body and breath. Place your hands on your belly.

Now inhale to a count of two, expanding your belly. Pause for a count of four. Then slowly exhale to a count of six. Each time you exhale, consciously relax your muscles and release tension from your brain and body.

Try a few cycles and see how you feel. Five to 10 cycles of 2:4:6 breathing is ideal.

Completed! [   ]

Day 7. Your Movement Practice

The most powerful stimulus for mitogenesis and positive mito-plasticity is movement. Therefore, the foundation of your mito-chondrial challenge is consistent movement. But I don't want you to think of movement as a workout. This is simply a practice.

The key is that when we think of movement as a practice it takes a lot of the stress and pressure away. It helps us think of movement as something we will slowly but consistently get better at.

So today I would love you to do a movement practice you enjoy for about 30 minutes. You can go longer if you want, but choose something you can do consistently, easily. If you are already prac-tising movement every day, try something new and be deliberate.

Go for a walk, take a yoga class, ride your bike, lift some weights, do some gardening, or do anything else you enjoy. We will do this every seventh day.

Remember that you can track your workouts on our VIIVIO app (download at www.viiv.io).

Completed! [   ]

Day 8. One Thing in the Morning

As you begin your second week in this challenge, consider instill-ing one healthy habit into your morning routine.

Consider what is most important to you right now.

Is it practising mindfulness? In that case, perhaps you want to brush your teeth with your non-dominant hand.

Is it gratitude? Then set a reminder in your calendar for each day this week to send a quick thank-you note.

Is it exercise? Then in the morning add a few minutes of move-ment to begin your day. You can stretch, go for a swim, walk or cycle, or even lift a few weights. Break a sweat and you win.

You can also pick anything you enjoyed practising from the previous week. Win your morning and you will win your day.

Completed! [   ]

Day 9. Practise Belly Breathing

Today, practise some belly breathing, ideally when you are feeling tired, stressed, or anxious.

To begin, get in a relaxed position or lie faceup with one hand on your navel.

As you inhale, expand your belly, pulling more air down into the lower part of the lungs. Your hand should rise as your belly expands. It's okay to expand your belly like a baby or like a statue of a Buddha.

As you exhale, contract your belly and push the air out so your hand falls and your belly returns to a resting position.

Doing this a few times throughout the day will help bring your attention to your breath, help you release mental and physical tension, and lower stress and anxiety.

Completed! [   ]

Day 10. Try Yoga

Yoga is an ancient practice that flows through a series of movements and poses to improve strength, flexibility, and balance. Although there are many different types of practices, all types of yoga focus on bringing the attention to the breath.

If you are already practising, that's great. Just do an intentional practice today. If you are new to yoga, give it a try. Remember that it's not about being good or bad at yoga. Simply practising is so wonderful for you.

Take a class at a local studio. Give them a call, just mention you are interested in getting started, and see what classes they recommend for you to try.

If you want to practise at home (I do), you can try a YouTube yoga class. I like Yoga with Adriene: www.youtube.com/c/yogawithadriene. You can also use Apple Fitness+ on your iPhone, which has great yoga classes, and Pocket Yoga is a good app for Android. And you might want to consider getting a yoga mat and some blocks.

Yoga and walking are the two key activities that, if practised consistently, can elevate your health and wellbeing throughout your entire life. It also does not matter where you are on the spectrum of fitness and even whether you have never exercised before.

Completed! [   ]

Day 11. Get a Water Container

Other than oxygen, water is the next most important substance that we need for life. Our bodies are 70% water. Remember that water powers the chemical pathways in our mitochondria that break down the food we eat to create the energy we use to power our lives.

So today make drinking water easier. Get a container that you can put in your refrigerator to keep your water cool. You can use tap water of course, but I like filtered water that is cold.

I also have glass containers that I fill with water and place on my desk. When I have water within reach, I tend to sip all day. If the containers are not there I forget.

So today's challenge is to get some containers for your water, fill them up, and place them in your fridge and on your desk.

Completed! [   ]

Day 12. Call a Friend

We know that social connections are one of the most powerful influences on our health and wellbeing. Social connections can be cultivated. Consider yourself the gardener of your social relationships.

So today connect with someone positive in your life. But let's go beyond a simple SMS or DM on social. Send a voice memo. Call them. Be prepared though—if you call someone they may pick up in a panic and ask, "What's wrong?" That is how rare actual direct conversation has become.

Don't feel like talking to someone? No worries. Listen to an awesome podcast or audiobook. That's a great way to have a "conversation" with some of the most brilliant minds in our world and history.

Completed! [   ]

Day 13. Practise Belly Breathing

Belly breathing is a very effective strategy to bring your attention into the present moment and to your breath and to calm your mind and body down.

As you did earlier in this challenge, sit in a relaxed position or lie faceup with one hand on your navel.

As you inhale, expand your belly, pulling more air down into the lower part of the lungs. Your hand should rise as your belly expands.

As you exhale, contract your belly and push the air out so your hand falls and your belly returns to a resting position. Take 10 slow, deep, relaxing belly breaths.

Completed! [   ]

Day 14. Your Movement Practice

The most powerful stimulus for mitogenesis and positive mito-plasticity is movement. Remember, the foundation of your mitochondrial challenge is consistent movement, and this is a practice. This is your weekly movement consistency day.

When we think of movement as a practice, it takes the pressure away and helps us think of movement as something we are consistently getting better at.

Today I would love you to do a movement practice you enjoy for about 30 minutes. You can go longer if you want, but choose something you can do consistently, easily.

Go for a walk, take a yoga class, ride your bike, lift some weights, do some gardening, or do anything else you enjoy. If you are already practising movement every day, try something new and be deliberate.

Completed! [   ]

Day 15. One Thing in the Evening

As you begin your third week in this challenge, consider instilling one healthy habit into your *evening* routine. Hopefully if this proves a meaningful addition to your life, it will become one of your treasured daily rituals.

Consider how you can best unwind from your day.

Perhaps you can put your phone away earlier and not check it in the hour before bed.

Perhaps you can take a bath to decompress and relax.

Perhaps you can write down five things you are grateful for in your journal.

Perhaps you can read a story to your kids and really be there with them 100%.

You can also pick anything you enjoyed practising from the previous week. We set ourselves up for a deep and restful sleep by downshifting positively at the end of the day.

Let's add that new ritual to the end of each of your days this week.

Completed! [   ]

Day 16. Box Breathing

In stressful situations, staying calm, cool, and collected can make all the difference between positive and negative outcomes. Practise box breathing for a few minutes.

When you are ready, breathe in, counting to four. Hold your breath for four counts. Exhale, counting to four. Hold your breath for four counts. This helps keep the sympathetic (stress and perform) nervous system and parasympathetic (rest and recover) nervous system in balance.

This simple tactic can help you do what you need to do at the highest level under the most challenging conditions so you can respond to the pressure rather than simply react to the situation. Try it the next time you're feeling nervous about something you need to do, and watch your nervous system calm down and your mind settle and relax.

Completed! [   ]

Day 17. Try Tai Chi or Qigong

Tai chi and qigong are martial arts that are popular practices for relieving stress and improving health. They both involve performing a series of flowing movements while focusing on the breath and being in the present moment.

You can register for an introductory class in your neighbourhood or at a gym near your workplace (if you are lucky enough to have one close by).

You can check out Taiflow, Dr. Paul Lam, or Peter Chen on YouTube for some videos on how to get started learning tai chi or qigong.

Keep an open mind, and don't take yourself too seriously. I learned tai chi with my friend and epic personal trainer Adrian Li while in Portugal on a trip a few years ago. It is a practice I love to use when I am tired or have had a tough day and I just don't want to go for a run or do a strenuous workout.

This practice always makes me feel better after I do it. Try it and let me know what you think.

Completed! [   ]

Day 18. Take a Cold Shower

Wait. Don't give up on the challenge. Cold water is soooo good for you.

When you have your shower today, wash your hair, soap your body, rinse off, and take a moment to breathe. Direct the flow of water to your forehead or to the space at the base of your neck between your shoulder blades.

Rest and relax for a minute. Just breathe. Then turn the temperature down. Just make the water cool to cold. Allow the cool water to cascade over your forehead or shoulders. Breathe.

We are looking for about 30 seconds. So you can count to 30 (as fast or slow as you want). Then turn the shower off and you can start your day powered up and energized, knowing you have already accomplished something really challenging.

Completed! [   ]

Day 19. Practise Gratitude

Today, simply think about what you are grateful for.

At home we ask the following questions around the dinner table, which I learned from my friends Bart Egnal and Emily Mather:

"What went well? What was hard? What are you looking forward to?"

You can also just list five things you are grateful for:

1. I am grateful for:
2. I am grateful for:
3. I am grateful for:
4. I am grateful for:
5. I am grateful for:

Judith does this daily with our kids right before we all go to sleep.

Completed! [   ]

Day 20. Drink Half Your Body Weight in Water

Drink half of your body weight (in pounds) in ounces of water each day, but especially today.

This means a 150-pound adult needs 75 ounces of water, or approximately nine cups. A 200-pound adult needs 100 ounces of water, or approximately 12 cups.

A lot of people aren't properly hydrated because they find the taste of water boring. If this is you, try adding a squirt of lemon juice to your glass of water. Not only will it add some flavour to the drink, but it also promotes hydration, helps with digestion, and gives you a boost of antioxidants.

You can keep track of your hydration in our VIIVIO app (download at www.viiv.io).

Completed! [   ]

Day 21. Your Movement Practice

Remember, the foundation of your mitochondrial challenge is consistent movement, and this is a practice. This is your weekly movement consistency day.

Today I would love you to do a movement practice you enjoy for about 30 minutes. You can go longer if you want, but choose something you can do consistently, easily.

Go for a walk, take a yoga class, ride your bike, lift some weights, do some gardening, or do anything else you enjoy. If you are already practising movement every day, try something new and be deliberate.

Completed! [   ]

Day 22. One Thing during the Day

As you begin your fourth week in this 100-day challenge, I would like you to consider instilling one healthy habit in your *daytime* routine. Hopefully if this proves a meaningful addition to your life, it will become one of your treasured daily rituals.

Consider how you can best perform during your day at work or at school.

Can you go for a quick walk during the day to recharge?

Can you do a few breaths and bring your attention to the present moment for two minutes at 2 p.m.?

Can you review your goals and make sure your daily actions are in alignment with your dreams?

Can you pack or order a healthy lunch with protein, veggies, and healthy fats?

You can also pick anything you enjoyed practising from the previous week. We set ourselves up for world-class performance by deliberately instilling practices that bring us energy during the day.

Let's add that new ritual to each of your days this week.

Completed! [   ]

Day 23. Have Some Yogic Coffee

Try the bellows breath, also known as the stimulating breath, instead of a cup of coffee today.

Sit comfortably with good posture and take a few deep breaths. Consciously relax your body and bring your attention to the here and now. Allow your mind to settle and quiet. Bring your attention to your breath.

Inhale and exhale through your nose, keeping your mouth closed and relaxed for a few breaths. Use your diaphragm to inhale and exhale, keeping your rib cage muscles relaxed.

Now inhale and exhale through your nose quickly (keeping your mouth closed). Aim for one to two cycles per second. Try this for five breath cycles, and then return to natural, gentle breathing. Observe your mindset.

As you practise, you can gradually build your blocks of breathing from 15 seconds up to 60 seconds. Give yourself two to three minutes of recovery between efforts.

Make sure to listen to your body as you do this practice. You are hyperventilating for short periods of time, so you might feel light-headed as you blow off carbon dioxide from your blood and lungs. If you experience this sensation, simply pause your practice and return to natural breathing for a few minutes until the discomfort passes. When you try again, experiment with slower bellows breathing with less intensity.

Completed! [   ]

Day 24. Break a Sweat

Today you are going to do some exercise that is a bit more challenging. I just want you to break a sweat. If you don't sweat much naturally, then you can just dress warmly and use your clothing to help increase blood flow.

You have a host of options today. Go for a walk but speed up a bit. Walk up a hill. Do some yoga. Ride your bike. Lift some weights. Clean the house (vacuuming works well). Go to the park with your kids and play. You are looking for anything physical that results in increased blood flow and breathing rate. Just break a sweat.

Completed! [   ]

Day 25. Get Some Sun

We know that sunlight has a host of benefits for our physiology and psychology. Just 5 to 15 minutes of sunscreen-free sunlight exposure at around midday, several times a week, is sufficient for your body to produce enough vitamin D without getting a sunburn. Sunlight is a hormetic agent, so a little is good but a lot is damaging. As always, practise moderation.

Go outside and get some exposure to natural light. Find a park bench in the sun and sit and enjoy the warmth of our closest star. If it's cloudy out, that is totally okay—natural light, even in cloudy conditions, is helpful.

You are looking for 5 to 15 minutes of outdoor light exposure today. That's it. Avoid prolonged exposure and sunburn, check that sun exposure is okay if you're taking any medicine, and check with your doctor or dermatologist to ensure that short outdoor sun exposures are safe for you.

Completed! [   ]

Day 26. Be Mindful, Young Padawan

In *Star Wars*, the Jedi Masters always remind the young Jedis who are in training (the Padawan learners) to "be mindful." So we can all channel our inner Jedi and practise a little mindful breathing today.

Sit, stand, or lie down in a comfortable place where you can focus completely for a few minutes. Relax and bring your attention to your breath.

Take a few breaths and simply notice them passing by. Each breath will be slightly different.

Now count your breaths as they pass. You can count one on the inhale and two on the exhale, then three on the inhale and four on the exhale. You can choose to count to 10 and then start over at one, which helps keep the mind from wandering.

If you do notice that your mind has wandered, you can start back at one. Starting over at one can be done non-judgmentally. You simply notice that your mind has wandered, gently invite your attention back to your breath, and begin counting again.

Completed! [   ]

Day 27. Let's Have Some Fun

As I discussed in the Thrive section of the book, so many of us have forgotten how to have fun. Kids know how to have fun intuitively. It's part of our nature as humans. But we got busy. Let's shake it up and bring more fun into our lives.

Today's task is to list five things that are fun for you.

Fun thing #1:

Fun thing #2:

Fun thing #3:

Fun thing #4:

Fun thing #5:

Awareness leads to clarity and clarity leads to life mastery.

Share this list with someone you love. Or post it on social and tag me @drgregwells.

Completed! [   ]

Day 28. Your Movement Practice

Remember, the foundation of your mitochondrial challenge is consistent movement, and this is a practice. This is your weekly movement consistency day.

Today I would love you to do a movement practice you enjoy for about 45 minutes. We are increasing the time duration this week from 30 minutes to 45.

Go for a walk, take a yoga class, ride your bike, lift some weights, do some gardening, or do anything else you enjoy. If you are already practising movement every day, try something new and be deliberate.

Completed! [   ]

Day 29. My Three Wins

If you are on day 29 of a 100-day challenge, and tens of thousands of words into a book on health, wellbeing, and self-improvement, then you are a very high performer. You rock. You are awesome.

One of the challenges of being a high performer who is awesome, however, is that you are probably always looking forward, planning, dreaming, and goal setting your way to a great life. Although this is a great strength, we often don't pause to give ourselves credit for how far we have come.

When we look back on our accomplishments and deliberately acknowledge and celebrate them, we build our confidence that we can continue to make progress and overcome any challenge we are faced with.

So today I would like you to look back over the last month of the 100-day challenge and give yourself credit for three things you added to your life that were positive. You only need to have tried three things and you win today's daily challenge.

My win #1:

My win #2:

My win #3:

Ping me with your awesomeness @drgregwells on Instagram or Twitter.

Completed! [   ]

Day 30. The Breath of Fire

Today is the first really challenging practice I am going to ask you to do on the 100-day mitochondrial makeover.

The breath of fire involves imagining a flame moving up and down your spine as you breathe.

Sit comfortably with good posture and take a few deep breaths. Consciously relax your body and bring your attention to the here and now. Allow your mind to settle and quiet. Close your eyes.

Take a few moments to visualize a flame in the air just in front of your body. Now enclose that flame in a hollow balloon, with the ball of fire inside the balloon. Imagine bringing the fire inside your belly.

Keep this image active throughout the practice. When your mind wanders, gently bring your attention back to the fire.

Place your hands on your stomach so you can feel your breath of fire throughout your abdomen.

Keep visualizing the internal fire, breathing smoothly and slowly as you feel the heat in your belly.

Invite the imaginary flame to move up your spine as you inhale and down your spine as you exhale.

Practise this for five to 10 slow, deep, relaxing breaths.

Bring your attention back to your physical body and the environment around you. Open your eyes and enjoy the energy, heat, and mental activation.

This technique is great to do in the morning, before a workout, or before an important event like a big presentation. Don't try this one before going to sleep.

Completed! [   ]

Day 31. Flex Your Mitochondrial Muscles

Today you will be putting a bit of action into your muscles. While cardio and aerobic exercise is incredible for your heart, lungs, and blood, your muscles thrive on resistance exercise. Simply put, I want you to put your muscles under some load so they are stimulated to grow and get stronger. With more muscle fibre comes more mitochondria.

Here are some ideas of activities that are considered muscle-building resistance activities.

Swimming. Swimming is predominantly an aerobic activity, but it also strengthens your muscles because you exert force against the water each time you take a stroke.

Paddling. Like swimming, workouts such as canoeing, kayaking, rowing, and stand-up paddleboarding require that you exert force against the water each time you take a stroke.

Skiing and snowboarding. These fun winter activities can provide another sneaky strength workout. Skiing and snowboarding require a lot of strength and stability.

Pilates. Pilates is a guided workout that combines strength, balance, and flexibility. Its focus is on the core muscles to improve posture, alleviate pain, and prevent injuries. Find a nearby studio or online class to guide you through a practice.

Weights. The most classic type of strength training can also be done at home or at a gym using simple weights like dumbbells or machines. If you need some help getting started, book a time with an instructor to make sure you are doing your exercises with good technique. One session with your trainer pays off for months.

Completed! [   ]

Day 32. Direct Your Energy to What You Can Control

The wonderful thing about sparking new and more powerful mitochondria is that you will have more energy. The challenge, once you have more energy, is to deliberately direct your energy to the areas of your life where you want it to go. Remember that where your attention goes, your energy flows.

To that end, direct your attention to what you can control and ignore what you cannot. Champion snowboarder Lindsey Jacobellis focuses on the small things she can do to prepare, such as getting her equipment ready and focusing the night before a competition. She doesn't waste time worrying about uncontrollable variables like how her competitors looked in training. These strategies help athletes feel as though they have a degree of control over the situation and allow them to overcome the feelings of being anxious and overwhelmed.

So let's make a list of three things in your life that would benefit from your attention and energy.

1.

2.

3.

Now deliberately and intentionally try to direct your attention and energy to the highest priorities in your life that you can positively influence.

Completed! [   ]

Day 33. Don't Worry, Be Happy

Today we are shifting our perspective on happiness. Remember, don't confuse seeking happiness with trying to be happy all the time. In fact, trying to be happy all the time makes us less happy, because we're constantly chasing (and failing to achieve) an unrealistic expectation.

Today, focus on creating happy moments when you can, and accepting the lows as they come as well.

Tell a joke, laugh for no reason, note something you are grateful for, smile at your partner (or a stranger), or do something you love (like riding your bike).

Consider this daily challenge completed when you can think of at least one little thing that you did, or that happened to you, that sparked a bit of happiness in your day. Bonus points if you managed to do this for someone else as well.

Completed! [   ]

Day 34. The Transition Ritual

One of the top five blog posts I have ever posted on www.drgregwells.com/blog has to do with the idea of adding a transition ritual to your day.

To live a high-performance life and do your best work, it is important to draw healthy boundaries between work and your home life. With technology making us so accessible, we run the risk of never detaching from work, especially if we work from home.

Therefore, we recommend instilling a transition ritual between work time and home time. This means starting and finishing your day with intention so you're not letting your work seep into your personal life, and vice versa.

Create a ritual that tells you it's either time for work or time for home. This will help cue your body and mind for work and focus or for rest and relaxation.

For example, maybe you like going for a walk outside in the morning and evening to emulate a "commute" to work. Or maybe once you get to your desk in the morning, you like to meditate for two minutes. Or once you're done work, you make sure to change out of your work clothes right away before doing anything else (even if you work from home this practice can be a very powerful way to distinguish between work and home life).

Remember, repetition is key. Switching your energy from "work" to "home" takes some upfront effort. But over time, cueing your brain in this way makes the shift easier and easier. It becomes automatic, so you can enter your personal time stress-free rather than mentally carrying your work items into your home life.

To complete today's challenge, simply practise any deliberate ritual that separates work from home activities.

Completed! [   ]

Day 35. Your Movement Practice

Remember, the foundation of your mitochondrial challenge is consistent movement, and this is a practice. This is your weekly movement consistency day.

Today I would love you to do a movement practice you enjoy for about 45 minutes. You can go longer if you want, but choose something you can do consistently, easily.

Go for a walk, take a yoga class, ride your bike, lift some weights, do some gardening, or do anything else you enjoy. This is your fifth week—you are doing great.

Completed! [   ]

Day 36. Take an Hour Off Technology

Another powerful way to decrease stress and to perform better more consistently is to take some time to unplug.

In today's world of the internet and smart phones and watches, we're constantly being bombarded with phone calls, messages, and news. It's important to step away from technology and be fully unplugged occasionally.

Today's challenge is to leave your phone at home or at the office and go for a walk and just enjoy being disconnected. The goal is one hour per day of no-device time.

This small dose of device-free time will leave you feeling refreshed and will ease some of your psychological stress.

The challenge is to try this today, but more importantly to determine what your device-free hour is going to be each day moving forward. Build this thrive time into your schedule.

Completed! [   ]

Day 37. Alternate Nostril Breathing

One type of breathing practice that is fantastic for bringing your attention into the present moment is alternate nostril breathing. I find it helpful for centring my mind and helping me be aware of my internal physiology.

In this very simple technique, you simply inhale and exhale through one nostril at a time. Here's how it works.

Sit, stand, or lie down in a comfortable place where you can focus completely for a few minutes. Bring your right hand up to just in front of your face. Gently place your pointer and middle fingertips against your forehead, right on or above your eyebrows, and use them as an anchor.

Bring your right thumb to your right nostril. With your right nostril closed, gently close your eyes and exhale slowly and completely through your left nostril, then inhale slowly and completely through the left nostril.

Release your thumb from the right nostril, and then use your ring finger to gently close your left nostril. With your left nostril closed, exhale slowly and completely through your right nostril, then inhale slowly and completely through the right nostril.

You can pause briefly at the end of your inhale and at the end of your exhale. Swap nostrils at the end of your inhales.

A smooth, consistent pattern is helpful for nostril breathing. You can try a 4-2-4-2 pattern: exhale for a count of four, pause for a count of two, inhale for a count of four, pause for a count of two (switch nostrils here at the end of your inhale).

Repeat the cycle five to 10 times, allowing your mind to follow the inhales and exhales. Practise a little smile, and then open your eyes and give yourself some props for doing your breath session.

Completed! [   ]

Day 38. Move Outside

It's time to practise some shinrin-yoku, or nature medicine. Please get out of your apartment, condo, house, school, or office. Spend some time outside. Ideally in a park, near some trees, or on a beach near water. If you live in a city and there are no parks that are easily accessible, that's totally okay. Just get out of the built structures.

Go for an easy walk, find a park bench to chill out on, sit on the beach and stare at the waves, look at some trees (hug them even?). Proximity to plants is what you are looking for. If you can add water that is even better. Remember the green workout and blue workout concepts? That is what you are seeking right now, but without the workout. ☺

There is no timeline for this one. Give yourself as much time as you want in the outdoors. Five minutes is awesome; 90 minutes is brilliant. It all helps.

Completed! [   ]

Day 39. Defend Your Sleep

This is a tough one. But the payoff is huge. I need you to commit to keeping your phone and tablet out of the bedroom before sleep. **More specifically, don't bring your phone into your bedroom.** Set up a charging station in another part of the house.

Researchers have found that children who used media devices

before bed had an increased likelihood of inadequate sleep, poor sleep quality, and excessive daytime sleepiness.

The same is true for adults, where even having the device in the room was associated with detrimental sleep effects, which is why it's important to not even bring your phone into the bedroom.

Invest in an alarm clock and use that to wake yourself up instead. This is your challenge. Get an alarm clock. Commit to no more tech right before you sleep. Note that you can track your sleep using our VIIVIO app (download at www.viiv.io).

Completed! [   ]

Day 40. Give Yourself a Day to Unplug

This is a big one.

In today's world we're constantly being bombarded with phone calls, messages, and news. It's important to step away from technology and be fully unplugged occasionally.

Leave your phone at home and go for a walk or hike and just enjoy being disconnected. This small dose of device-free time will leave you feeling refreshed and will ease some of your psychological stress.

Today you are practising taking an entire day without your devices. If you need to do this on a weekend that is totally fine, but I challenge you to try it on a weekday.

A couple of years ago I dropped my phone in Lake Ontario while out paddleboarding. I was so stressed that I would miss work calls or not be able to check email on the go.

It took a few days to get a new phone and get it set up. Those were three glorious days. I gradually noticed my attention returning to the present, and I let go of the need to constantly check my notifications.

The world will survive without you constantly checking your device for a day.

Completed! [   ]

Day 41. Have a Berry Blast Smoothie

Berry Blast Smoothie

Add 1 cup baby spinach to a blender with ¼ cup water and blend until smooth.

Add the following ingredients to the blended spinach

- ¼ avocado
- ½ banana
- ½ cup blueberries (or blackberries)
- 1 tbsp ground flaxseeds
- 1 tsp cinnamon
- 1 scoop vegan protein powder (I like LivingFuel LivingProtein)
- 1 cup (or more) unsweetened coconut milk.

Blend and enjoy.

PS: For other great smoothie recipes, check out *The Plantpower Way* by Rich Roll and *Oh She Glows* by Angela Liddon. If you have a favourite healthy smoothie recipe, share it with me @drgregwells so we can uplevel the community.

Completed! [   ]

Day 42. Your Movement Practice

Remember, the foundation of your mitochondrial challenge is consistent movement, and this is a practice. This is your weekly movement consistency day.

Today I would love you to do a movement practice you enjoy for about 45 minutes. You can go longer if you want, but choose something you can do consistently, easily.

Go for a walk, take a yoga class, ride your bike, lift some weights, do some gardening, or do anything else you enjoy.

Completed! [   ]

Day 43. Clean Out Your Kitchen

My friend and colleague Dr. John Berardi from Precision Nutrition has a simple saying. He suggests that "if a food is in your home, you or someone you love will eventually eat it." So today I challenge you to make success inevitable.

Make it easy to eat healthy—especially when you are tired and stressed. How can you do this? By having healthy food and especially healthy snacks that are ready to go at all times. I like berries, nuts, and veggies and hummus as my go-tos.

But even more important than having the healthy food on hand is to make eating unhealthy foods more difficult. Which means getting them out of your kitchen, pantry, and home.

I hate wasting food, but it's best for all of humanity that you throw out the food that no longer serves you.

Junk food, fast food, as well as refined carbohydrates including white pasta, soft drinks, white bread, and many breakfast cereals can all go.

It's okay to have a treat occasionally. Just go out for treats, rather than keeping them readily available at home and at work.

Completed! [   ]

Day 44. The Reset Breath

Here's a technique to help sharpen your concentration and attention at work or while studying.

Sit in your chair and place both feet on the floor. Sit up tall. Bring your attention to your body and breath. Place your hands on your belly.

Now inhale to a count of two and lean upward as you expand your belly.

Look to the sky as you pause for a count of three. Add a little smile as you look to the sky.

Then slowly exhale and curl forward, and keep exhaling until you are out of breath. Each time you exhale, consciously relax your muscles and release tension from your brain and body.

Once you have the pattern set, close your eyes, and repeat this cycle five to 10 times.

Completed! [   ]

Day 45. Go for an "Awe Walk"

A hike through a sublime mountain range often creates feelings of awe—admiration, wonder, even a sense of being a small speck in a vast universe—but an everyday walk can also become an "awe walk."

During an ordinary awe walk, you would pay attention to the small wonders around you. The leaves on the trees. The daisies in a garden. A small dog rolling on the grass. An awe walk combines walking, which is already healthy and boosts your mood, with an intentional focus on the beautiful elements of your environment. Awe involves getting out of your own head to notice and admire what's around you.

It's good to get out of your head and connect to the beauty and wonder of the world.

You can walk indoors or outdoors. I always encourage getting outside in nature for the extra health benefits, but the great thing about walking is you can pretty much do it anywhere. Just avoid crowded places like the mall around holidays. No knocking other people over on your quest for brain health.

Keep checking in to ensure you're in the here and now. When you notice your mind wandering, just gently bring your attention back to the present and the cool and interesting things in your immediate environment

Completed! [   ]

Day 46. Get Some Blue Exercise

Today I want you to go for a swim. If swimming is not your thing, then aquafit is also great. Any sort of paddling, like stand-up paddleboarding, also works.

You can also just go for a walk near a river, lake, or ocean. If none of these are available, just take a bath and splash around like a little kid and laugh and have fun.

Blue exercise creates something called "blue mind." Simply, you want to exercise in or near bodies of water, like lakes, rivers, oceans, or indoor or outdoor pools.

Blue mind as a result of being physically close to water—like being by a lake—yields a state of increased calm and wellness, better sleep, and decreased stress and anxiety.

And as you now know, anything that lowers stress and anxiety sparks your mitochondria.

Completed! [   ]

Day 47. Take a Sauna

It's time to practise heat exposure again. Saunas are great—both infrared saunas and traditional saunas are fine. Hot showers work, and hot baths are equally fantastic.

Sauna bathing induces mild hyperthermia from exposure to temperatures ranging from 45 °C to 100 °C. In fact, the physiological response following a trip to the sauna is comparable to that of exercise, providing a great alternative if you have trouble exercising or just don't have time on a given day.

Heat exposure like saunas and hot baths also offers protection against various cardiovascular diseases, reduces inflammation, enhances cognitive and mental health, increases your cardiorespiratory fitness, and preserves muscle mass via mitogenesis.

Today I'd like you to aim for a 5- to 10-minute-long hot bath or shower or a 10- to 20-minute-long sauna.

Completed! [   ]

Day 48. Count Your Breaths

Bringing your attention to your breath has the physiological effect of lowering your heart rate and blood pressure while reducing feelings of burnout, exhaustion, and fatigue.

In addition to simply bringing your attention to the breath to gain these benefits, you can also use counting as an anchor for your mind.

Sit, stand, or lie down in a comfortable place where you can focus completely for a few minutes. Relax and bring your attention to your breath.

Take a few breaths and simply notice them passing by. Each breath will be slightly different.

Now count your breaths as they pass. You can count one on the inhale and two on the exhale, then three on the inhale and four on the exhale. You can choose to count to 10 and then start over at one, which helps keep the mind from wandering.

If you do notice that your mind has wandered, you can start back at one. Starting over at one can be done non-judgmentally. You simply notice that your mind has wandered, gently invite your attention back to your breath, and begin counting again.

It helps to set a timer for this exercise so you don't need to worry about counting cycles—you just practise for a set amount of time. Sessions of 3, 5, or 10 minutes work well.

Completed! [   ]

Day 49. Your movement practice

Remember, the foundation of your mitochondrial challenge is consistent movement, and this is a practice. This is your weekly movement consistency day.

Today I would love you to do a movement practice you enjoy for about 45 minutes. You can go longer if you want, but choose something you can do consistently, easily. If you are already practising movement every day, try something new and be deliberate.

Go for a walk, take a yoga class, ride your bike, lift some weights, do some gardening, or do anything else you enjoy.

Completed! [   ]

Day 50. My Three Wins

Day 50 of a 100-day challenge means you are halfway done. Congratulations!

Remember that when we look back on our accomplishments and deliberately acknowledge and celebrate them, we build our confidence that we can continue to make progress and overcome any challenge we are faced with.

So today I would like you to look back over the first half of the 100-day challenge and give yourself credit for three things you added to your life that were positive. You only need to have tried three things and you win today's daily challenge.

My win #1:

My win #2:

My win #3:

Ping me with your awesomeness @drgregwells on Instagram or Twitter.

Completed! [   ]

Day 51. Sync Your Breath and Movement

Today I would like you to practise a rhythmic movement activity like walking, jogging, running, cycling, or paddling. Flow yoga can also work.

As you do the activity at a comfortable but consistent pace, bring your attention to your breath as you are moving. The goal is to have your breathing in rhythm with your movement. If you are walking, breathe in for a couple of steps and out for a couple of steps. The same idea applies to all rhythm-based activities.

In flow yoga bring your attention to your breath, and use the deep inhales and exhales to flow through the movement patterns. The sun salutation sequence is perfect for learning this.

You will notice that your breathing, when nice and relaxed and entrained to the movement, can make the exercise feel easier. When your breathing is out of sync the movement will feel harder.

This moving meditation practice is great for your mind and

body. You can do this anytime to bring energy and focus to your day.

Completed! [   ]

Day 52. The Green Workout

Today you are looking to add 12 to 15 minutes of forest or park activity to your day. Even the busiest of us can spare 15 minutes once a day to get outside, whether to a local park or somewhere in the countryside.

Go for a walk in the park, do some yoga in your backyard, or do some gardening. Anything counts—the goal is to get some exercise while being exposed to plants.

I have often taken my kids to the playground, and while they play on the structures, I will do some stretches on the park bench or chase them around to keep them entertained.

You can do this before work or school as a mental boost, during the workday to decrease your stress, or at the end of the day as a transition ritual. After dinner is also awesome as a mental end-of-day relaxation activity.

Completed! [   ]

Day 53. Psych Up

We all have important events in our lives. These can be races we are participating in, music performances, tests we write, presentations at work, or important calls we need to make.

We need to make sure that when these moments arise, we are energetically aligned and ready to perform. We need the mitochondria in our brains to be activated and creating ATP for our neurons so they can work their magic and spark our cognition.

To that end I would love you to choose one event today to get ready for, and then to deliberately elevate your energy output so you can do your best to perform when you need to. Here are the four steps:

1. Eliminate distractions.

2. Listen to music that pumps you up.

3. Activate your body (stretch or go for a walk).

4. Practise positive self-talk. Tell yourself exactly how awesome you are and how you are going to do on today's important task.

Completed! [   ]

Day 54. Journal Your Successes

I have had the great fortune to have met some incredible people over the years. One of the benefits of being a professional speaker is spending time in the green room getting ready for presentations and sharing the space with others who are also speaking at the conference.

At one event early in my career I had the chance to meet with Richard Branson. One of the takeaways from that meeting was that he always carries a journal with him so he can capture ideas in written form as they occur. Journalling is a common habit of the high performers I have chatted with over the years.

In Matthew McConaughey's *Greenlights*, he describes not just journalling about his challenges or difficulties or daily activities but making detailed notes about his successes too.

He makes extensive records of the times in his life when he is at his best. When he is performing to his true potential. When he has energy. When he is at his very peak as an actor. That way he can look back on the practices he was implementing when he was doing well.

So today, make some notes about how you were acting,

thinking, and feeling when you were performing at your best at a task that was meaningful to you. Keep these notes somewhere so you can access them in the future when you need a boost.

Completed! [   ]

Day 55. More Energy, Less Tension

I have a simple practice for you today.

When you notice your stress levels rise, you will sense that your breathing becomes shallow, and you might clench your jaw or tense your muscles.

Notice if this happens and take a moment to consciously relax your face, shoulders, hands, stomach muscles, back, legs, and feet. Beginning at your head and working down, scan your body and release tension each time you exhale.

Release tension and notice your energy levels rise.

Completed! [   ]

Day 56. Your Movement Practice

Remember, the foundation of your mitochondrial challenge is consistent movement, and this is a practice. This is your weekly movement consistency day.

Today I would love you to do a movement practice you enjoy for about 45 minutes. You can go longer if you want, but choose something you can do consistently, easily. If you are already practising movement every day, try something new and be deliberate.

Go for a walk, take a yoga class, ride your bike, lift some weights, do some gardening, or do anything else you enjoy.

Completed! [   ]

Day 57. Have a Plant-Based Meal

I am a big fan of both the Mediterranean diet and eating as plant-based as possible.

Today your challenge is to have a plant-based meal. Adding one plant-based meal per week to your plan can make a big difference to your health and the health of the planet. Here is a great recipe from Dr. Melissa Piercell:

Vegan Chickpea Curry

Cook a medium diced onion and 4 cloves of minced garlic in 1 tbsp coconut oil on medium heat for a few minutes.

Lower the heat to medium, then add 2 cups cubed butternut squash, 2 cups organic vegetable broth, 4 tbsp ground turmeric, 1 tbsp coriander, 1 tbsp cumin, and ½ tsp ground ginger.

Cook for 10 minutes (until squash is tender), then add 1 can (540 mL) rinsed chickpeas, 1 cup organic shelled edamame, 1 can (400 mL) coconut milk, and 2 cups baby spinach.

Cook for another 10 minutes and serve on a bed of cooked quinoa with chopped cilantro and lime wedges.

Completed! [   ]

Day 58. The Breath of Joy

Today let's try a simple technique called the breath of joy. Following this practice can release tensions and increase your natural life force, or "prana," thus both generating and opening yourself to receiving joy.

Here are the simple instructions:

1. Stand with your feet shoulder-width apart and arms at your sides.

2. Inhale to one-third of your lung capacity while you bring your arms up in front of your body to shoulder level, with palms facing each other.

3. Now inhale to two-thirds capacity and stretch your arms out to the sides, still at shoulder height.

4. Now inhale to full capacity and raise your arms over your head as if you're reaching for the sky.

5. Finally, exhale through your mouth as you lean forward and "take a bow," with your arms stretched out to the sides and slightly behind you. As you finish this motion and exhalation, smile, and laugh.

Repeat this sequence four more times, for five times in total. As you become more familiar and comfortable with the combination of breathing and movements, try closing your eyes through each sequence and focusing your mind on the energy you feel circulating through your body.

Completed! [   ]

Day 59. Move for FUN

Our lives are often busy and highly scheduled. Everything can feel like it's on a timeline and must be measured and purposeful. You might notice that given time and space, children are so good at just playing and being immersed in the moment. They can have fun so easily.

Today I would like you to do something just for fun. Put away the heart rate monitor and go for a run. Do some yoga and don't worry about technique or whether you are stretching enough.

Better yet, try dancing. Turn up the music, put on a learn-to-dance video, and have a laugh.

Today your challenge is simply to do something super fun and 100% purely for the joy of it.

Completed! [   ]

Day 60. Let's Get Hot Again

Heat is a powerful stimulus for your mitochondria to get healthier. When we take a hot bath or sauna, we spark heat shock proteins in our bodies that create all sorts of positive adaptations.

Today I'd like you to aim for a 5- to 10-minute-long hot bath or shower, or a 10- to 20-minute-long sauna. If you are lucky enough to live somewhere hot, you can go outside and get your sweat on.

Completed! [   ]

Day 61. Practise Small Acts of Disconnection

Let's get some of your time back for you. In an era of constant distraction, your ability to control your attention is a superpower. Please choose one of the following ideas to implement today to eliminate distractions and elevate your life.

Turn your phone off and put it away during mealtimes with family and/or co-workers.

Batch your email. Choose two times today to check and deal with email, and don't look at it outside of those times.

Turn off your notifications. Your attention is yours. Don't let others steal it from you. Turn off notifications on your mobile devices so that you can check your communications when you want to, not when others want you to.

For more information on this, check out power-up #2 in chapter 4.

Completed! [   ]

Day 62. Read Fiction before Bed

Healing, recovery, and recharging happen when we sleep. This is when our bodies and brains repair and regenerate. This is when we assemble amino acids from the proteins we eat to create new and more powerful mitochondria. Simply put, mitogenesis happens when we sleep.

So sleeping better is key. Falling asleep quickly and staying asleep is the game we want to be playing.

So today I'd like you to choose bedtime reading that will slow your mind.

My sleep protocol involves reading physical books or using a reader that doesn't emit light. I also avoid reading anything that will activate my brain. For me, that means reading fiction. For other people, that means reading non-fiction like a biography or a history book.

Whatever you choose, ensure it helps your mind unwind, gear down, and rest. Don't be lounging in bed reviewing your materials for the big meeting the next day.

If you don't have any hard-copy books, you can order a few to get started. Technology is amazing—your new books can be at your house the next day.

Completed! [   ]

Day 63. Your Movement Practice

Remember, the foundation of your mitochondrial challenge is consistent movement, and this is a practice. This is your weekly movement consistency day.

Today I would love you to do a movement practice you enjoy for about 45 minutes. You can go longer if you want, but choose something you can do consistently, easily. If you are already practising movement every day, try something new and be deliberate.

Go for a walk, take a yoga class, ride your bike, lift some weights, do some gardening, or do anything else you enjoy.

Completed! [   ]

Day 64. Have an Ultra-Healthy Dinner

Eating healthy food with family and friends is a joy on so many levels. When you add anti-inflammatory ingredients, you help your mitochondria as well. Here is one of our favourite meals:

Easy Wild Salmon and Asparagus

Place 4 portions of salmon on a parchment-lined cookie sheet.

Spread a thin coating (4 tbsp) of spicy mustard on the fish and sprinkle with fresh dill (2 tbsp).

Toss 2 cups trimmed asparagus with avocado oil, salt, and pepper. Arrange on the baking sheet with the salmon.

Bake for 12 minutes at 400 °F, and serve with lemon wedges and cauliflower rice.

Completed! [   ]

Day 65. SKY Breathing

SKY stands for Sudarshan Kriya yoga, and SKY breathing is a unique yogic breathing practice that makes use of a range of slow (calming) and rapid (stimulating) breaths.

There are three main steps to do in sequence, which means you will have varying breathing rates separated by periods of normal breathing.

Here is the sequence:*

* Zope, S.A., and R.A. Zope. "Sudarshan Kriya yoga: Breathing for health." *International Journal of Yoga* 6, no. 1 (January 2013): 4–10.

1. Ujjayi, or "victorious breath": This involves experiencing the conscious sensation of the breath touching the throat. This slow breath technique increases airway resistance during inspiration and expiration and controls airflow. Try four slow, deep breaths where you create resistance in the back of your throat on the exhale.

2. "Bellows breath": Air is rapidly inhaled and forcefully exhaled at a rate of 30 breaths per minute. It causes excitation followed by calmness. Try 10 deep but faster breaths. Stop if you feel dizzy.

3. Take a deep breath in and then say "om" during your prolonged exhale.

4. You can repeat this cycle a few times.

Completed! [   ]

Day 66. Wake Up Your Muscle Mitochondria

Resistance training is usually thought of for increasing your strength—and it certainly works for that. But the other benefit of challenging your muscles with exercise that is different from traditional cardio is sparking mitogenesis and mitoplasticity to make your entire muscle system work better, from the microscopic level right through to your biceps.

If you want to try a strength training workout, we have created an example for you here: https://wellsperformance.com/strength-circuit. Some other strength-building options are as follows:

Housework. Believe it or not, even housework can count toward strength training, depending on the task.

Hiking. Any walk in which you're gaining elevation or adjusting to varying ground can count toward strength training, as you're producing significantly greater force than during a walk on flat ground. Stairs work in the same way. Taking a break at home or the office by climbing up and down the stairs is a super simple and effective option.

Body-weight workouts. Here's another no-special-equipment option. Whether or not you have access to a gym, there are many exercises that can be done using only your body weight. You can also easily sprinkle in some body-weight exercises throughout the day. Whatever works for you with the equipment (your own self), space, and time that you have.

Weights. The most classic type of strength training can also be done at home or at a gym using simple weights like dumbbells or machines. Especially when using weights, it's a good idea to get advice from a certified personal trainer or registered kinesiologist before performing an exercise you've never done before.

Today, just do any type of strength or resistance training to keep moving forward on your 100-day challenge.

Completed! [   ]

Day 67. Cool Off

After yesterday's strength session you might be a little sore. No worries—today I have a solution for that. I want you to cool off.

Cold exposure improves antioxidant and anti-inflammatory

capacity; increases energy expenditure, metabolism, and recovery following exercise; and enhances cognition and mental health.

You can take a cold shower as we talked about earlier in the challenge, but if you want to step it up and take it to the next level, today you can try cold-water immersion (although the cold shower still gets you your challenge success for today).

A cold bath or an ice bath can be used for cold-water immersion (CWI)—though few of us have easy access to a lot of ice at short notice. Outdoor CWI options include swimming in the ocean, which can be cold throughout the year depending on location, and lake swimming works as well.

As mentioned already, if you are new to CWI you can start with a few minutes of cold shower time and work your way up. If you're feeling brave, try jumping in a cold bath, ocean, or lake.

Experts suggest taking cold-water showers or ice baths at home before trying outdoor CWI to allow your body to become accustomed to the physiological response. Be cautious when you are cold swimming outdoors, and never go alone.

Today's goal is a longer cold shower or a quick plunge in a cold bath or open water like a lake or the ocean. If you want to learn more and do a course on CWI, look up the Wim Hof Method.

Completed! [   ]

Day 68. Find Your People

I have a simple practice for you today, although it is one that can have a profound impact on your overall life energy.

I would like you to think about and identify the five people in your life who are powerful positive influences on you. Who brings you energy? Who makes you happy? Who elevates your life?

Let's list them here:

Positive person #1:

Positive person #2

Positive person #3:

Positive person #4:

Positive person #5:

Great. Now make a point to reach out to these people and have a call, go for a walk, or even set up a time to go for a meal. Bring more positive energy into your life from the epic people who bring you joy and happiness. I make this list and reach out to people every three months or so.

If you don't have five people you can reach out to right now, you can also download an audiobook from a great author and learn directly from them or check out a few podcasts with interviews of people who are awesome and have ideas that can make your life better.

Completed! [   ]

Day 69. Respect the Need for Darkness

Although technology can be a wonderful tool for humanity, there is a challenge in that we are constantly exposed to light both from the sun and from our devices.

This is an issue because when light hits your eyes, it sends a signal to your brain that it's daytime and to stop producing melatonin, the hormone that makes you feel sleepy, with the blue light from screens particularly bad.

One of the most effective ways to fall asleep quickly (and have a restful sleep) is to avoid exposing your eyes to bright light within the hour before you'd like to be asleep. I call this "defending your last hour."

Have an alarm set to go off every night one hour before you'd like to be asleep. In our home, my family creates a digital sunset every evening. All our lights are on dimmer switches. As we near bedtime the devices go away, and we dim the lights in the house.

The key idea here is to respect the power of darkness. Get your sunshine . . . and then turn off all the lights and drop those blackout shades. To win today's challenge, I would like you to create a digital sunset in your home to help you fall asleep and stay asleep better.

Completed! [   ]

Day 70. Your Movement Practice

Remember, the foundation of your mitochondrial challenge is consistent movement, and this is a practice. This is your weekly movement consistency day.

Today I would love you to do a movement practice you enjoy for about 45 minutes. You can go longer if you want, but choose something you can do consistently, easily. If you are already practising movement every day, try something new and be deliberate.

Go for a walk, take a yoga class, ride your bike, lift some weights, do some gardening, or do anything else you enjoy.

Completed! [   ]

Day 71. Find Your Sweet Spot

I have a simple practice for you today that builds on challenge day 68.

I would like you to think about and identify the five *places* in your life that have powerful positive influences on you. What environment do you love? Where can you go where you feel a boost of positivity?

This might be your place of worship, a room in your home, a special vacation spot, your cottage, a park near your home, or just a place where you feel relaxed and at ease with those you love.

Let's list them here:

Positive place #1:

Positive place #2

Positive place #3:

Positive place #4:

Positive place #5:

Now that you know where you feel your best, I encourage you to think about deliberately programming spending time in those locations. I know I write easily and well in a coffee shop near my home, so at least once a week I spend the morning there writing blogs or notes for books.

Feel free to take a pic of your special spot and share with me on social @drgregwells.

Completed! [   ]

Day 72. Breathe to Music

Matching breathing to great music you love can be a powerful tool to elevate your mood, sharpen your concentration, and bring you into a state of flow.

Begin by taking a few deep breaths and allowing yourself to enjoy long exhales as you relax physically, mentally, and emotionally.

Then choose a song or album that you love, that makes you happy, and that you know very well (i.e., you have listened to it many times before).

Bring your attention to your breath and to the feeling of air moving in and out of your nostrils and airways as you enjoy your awesome music.

After a song or two, you can move into an activity, task, or project that is meaningful to you as you leave the music playing in the background. Relaxation plus breathing plus music is a combination you can leverage to perform to your potential and get into flow so you can have peak experiences.

Completed! [   ]

Day 73. Try the Joy Workout

When we're happy, excited, and joyful, our body language reflects how we feel. We might lift our arms or jump in the air. But it also works the other way around. When we move our bodies in a certain way, we can change the way we think and feel. In fact, research has shown that happiness and a positive emotional state can be improved simply through movement and dance. What's more, even watching someone perform "happy movements" can make us feel happy and joyful.

This is the idea behind the Joy Workout that you will be practising today. Simply add a few of these movements to your day. Here's a simple list:

- Reaching your arms up
- Swaying from side to side
- Bouncing to a beat
- Spinning with arms outstretched
- Shaking your body
- Jumping

You can do these moves in any order, as quickly or as slowly as you like, as big or as small as you like, and of course you can add music that makes you feel good. Up-tempo songs seem to work well. You can also double up on the movements you really like and drop any that don't uplift you.

It's amazing that choosing specific movements, like throwing your arms up in the air, can create feelings of joy. Try making up a movement routine that works for you.

Completed! [   ]

Day 74. Create Your High-Energy Soundtrack

Music can elevate our lives in so many ways. Today I have a simple task for you to do to earn your challenge point.

Create a soundtrack for your workout. Pick your favourite high-energy songs and label this playlist so you can quickly access it when you want to exercise.

I have a playlist for weights, running, and general workouts. I change them up every few months, but once you have them set it's so easy to ensure you have the right music at the right time for those high-energy moments.

PS: I also use my workout playlists for commutes to work when I have big presentations or keynotes.

Completed! [   ]

Day 75. Find Your Pursuits

I have a simple practice for you today that builds on challenge days 68 and 71. First you found your people. Then you identified your places. The last piece of this lifestyle-engineering puzzle is to know what pursuits bring you joy.

I would like you to think about and identify the five pursuits in your life that you simply love to partake in.

So what do you love to do?

Let's list them here:

Positive pursuit #1:

Positive pursuit #2

Positive pursuit #3:

Positive pursuit #4:

Positive pursuit #5:

Now that you know what you love to do, make sure to plan to do these activities on a daily, weekly, monthly, and yearly basis. The challenge today is to simply make the list. Then it's all up to you to deliberately build these pursuits into your life.

Completed! [   ]

Day 76. The Do Not Do List

Today's challenge is a simple but powerful tactic. Now that you know the people, places, and pursuits you want to have more of in your life, you need to create some space. To that end I encourage you to think not so much about creating the to-do list that is so common, but a "do not do" list.

Think about what you are no longer going to do. What are you going to say no to from now on? Who might you want to spend less time with? Where do you not want to waste your time in the future? What activities no longer serve you?

This can be a painful exercise, and you may be confronted with some difficult decisions. But life is short, and you want to make sure you craft a life where you can thrive and have a positive impact on the world.

What are you going to *not* do from now on? Let's make that list and start to protect your time, effort, attention, and energy so you can direct them to those people, places, and pursuits that are meaningful for you moving forward.

By the way, if you want to keep this simple, the do not do list is also effective at work. It helps me stay focused on priorities and activities that move the needle forward, and it keeps me from falling into the busy-but-not-effective trap.

Completed! [ ]

Day 77. Your Movement Practice

Remember, the foundation of your mitochondrial challenge is consistent movement, and this is a practice. This is your weekly movement consistency day.

Today I would love you to do a movement practice you enjoy for about 45 minutes. You can go longer if you want, but choose something you can do consistently, easily. If you are already practising movement every day, try something new and be deliberate.

Go for a walk, take a yoga class, ride your bike, lift some weights, do some gardening, or do anything else you enjoy.

Completed! [ ]

Day 78. Craft Your Ikigai, Part 1

Remember, the state of ikigai is traditionally defined as that which gives your life meaning and purpose or, in other words, "what makes life worth living." So today you will start to think deeply about that question and build some structure around your ikigai so you can instill more of it in your daily life.

Ken Mogi's five pillars of ikigai begin with starting small. Today your challenge is to pay attention to the smallest details related to the elements of your life that are most meaningful to you.

If you have children, perhaps you can notice the fine details of their faces. They might think you are looking at them in a strange way, but that's okay. Just let them know they are fascinating to you, and you love them.

If your workouts are important to you, then you can notice the details of the movements. How do your muscles feel as you lift the weights? How does your breathing feel during your running intervals? Bring your attention into your body, and enjoy the process and experience of being active.

Today the challenge is to start small. Notice the details in the moment. When we are aware of the elements in our lives that are meaningful to us, we are deliberately crafting our experience of our own ikigai.

Completed! [   ]

Day 79. Take Three Deep Breaths

I'm taking you right back to basics and day 2 of the 100-day challenge. Today, just do a few deep belly breaths.

Place a hand on your belly (the one not holding this book). Next, inhale deeply and fill your belly with your breath. Pause. Then exhale slowly to the count of seven. Try that once more, and let the exhale be gentle and slow. Repeat this cycle a few times.

Congratulations! You just practised mindful breathing and, in the process, calmed down your nervous system.

The key moving forward is to use these three deep breaths to bring you a sense of calm when you are stressed or anxious. It's easy to do this when you are rested and chill. It is more challenging to do when you are having a difficult moment. But it is in these moments of challenge where the true power of this technique will reveal itself.

Completed! [   ]

Day 80. Move and Flow

Getting into flow takes practice, but the more often you do it, the easier it will be. If you choose a challenging, enjoyable activity and create the right environment, you will learn to enter flow more easily, not only during exercise but in all areas of life.

Flow is when we are energized, motivated, focused, happy, and able to perform at our best. Getting into flow when you are moving is an easy way to get a sense of this state so that you can enter flow when needed in other areas of your life, like when you are working on a project, studying, or spending time with loved ones.

Today I would like you to walk, jog, run, cycle, swim, or paddle. Anything rhythmic and repetitive. I would like you to plan on at least 20 minutes and up to 45 minutes. Just go out and move in a rhythmic pattern.

Once you are in a rhythm—for example, you have been walking for a few minutes—find an intensity that is comfortable and sustainable. Not easy and not too hard. Settle in and spend a few more minutes in that zone.

The next step is counterintuitive. I'd like you to let your mind wander and allow yourself to be distracted. Let your attention go where it wants. Practise non-judgment. Just walk (jog, swim, bike, or paddle) with an open, relaxed mind.

This state of gentle repetitive movement with an open and non-judgmental mind will often help people drop into a state where everything feels easy, and time seems to pass quickly.

It's also just a really nice way to enjoy some activity with a relaxed mindset. Give it a try and earn your challenge point.

Completed! [   ]

Day 81. Create Your Happy Mood Soundtrack

Music can elevate our lives in so many ways. Today I have a simple task for you to do to earn your challenge point.

I'd love you to create a soundtrack for the moments in your life when you want to be happy and relaxed. How you want to feel when you are driving home from work to see your family. How you want to feel during dinner with loved ones. How you want to feel on a chill weekend morning at home.

Pick your favourite happiness and joy songs, and label this playlist so you can quickly access it when you want to elevate your mood and create a happy space.

Judith has a playlist that she and the kids listen to on the way to school in the morning. She also has an epic '90s hip hop mix that is fantastic for dinner or when people come over.

Let's use music to create a happy, positive vibe in our homes and the places we share with those we love.

Completed! [   ]

Day 82. Craft Your Ikigai, Part 2

As we challenge ourselves to keep building a life of energy, health, and wellbeing, we want to make sure we are deliberately leveraging the power of crafting our ikigai. I have learned so much from Terry Stuart, the chief innovation officer at Deloitte Consulting, one of my favourite clients at Wells Performance. Terry is obsessed with exploring meaning and purpose.

Outside of his immediate role at Deloitte, Terry has focused his attention on the Awesome Music Project, or AMP (www .theawesomemusicproject.com). AMP uses music to help people with mental health challenges and organizes concerts to raise money to support mental health initiatives in the community. It's pretty awesome. Watching Terry talk about AMP is a great way to see someone light up when they are on mission. I want you to experience the same thing.

Today I want you to take 15 minutes (or more if you want) to practise life crafting. As explained in chapter 4 (Thrive), life crafting involves the following:

- Exploring your passions
- Knowing what you are good at and what brings you energy
- Spending time and attention on your relationships and social life
- Aligning your career and your mission where possible
- Practising goal setting related to the meaningful elements in your life

So today just spend 15 or more minutes on any of these ideas. Think about your mission. Plan some activities around your mission. Commit time, energy, and attention to your purpose.

Completed! [   ]

Day 83. Add Some Phytochemicals to Your Diet

Phytochemicals act as important antioxidants and induce hormesis—the adaptive stress-resistant process that makes our mitochondria stronger and healthier. The two most significant antioxidant-contributing phytochemicals found in plants and foods are polyphenols and carotenoids.

These phytochemicals are potent free-radical scavengers and anti-inflammatory agents. Polyphenols are the most prevalent natural antioxidants found in the human diet and can be found in wine, green tea, coffee, grapes, cherries, and chocolate.

Carotenoids are responsible for the orange, yellow, and red

colours of different foods and are found in vegetables and fruits including sweet potato, spinach, carrots, bell peppers, beans, and pumpkin.

So today's challenge is to add some phytochemicals to your diet. Any of the following will work:

- Have a glass of red wine.
- Drink some tea or coffee (skip the sugar and milk).
- Have a handful of fresh grapes or cherries.
- Eat some 70%+ cocoa or chocolate.
- Add some sweet red, yellow, or orange bell peppers to a salad.
- Have some beans with rice as a side with your dinner.
- Roast some sweet potatoes and have them as a side with lunch or dinner. Cinnamon or paprika make for great spices on sweet potato.

Completed! [   ]

Day 84. Your Movement Practice

Remember, the foundation of your mitochondrial challenge is consistent movement, and this is a practice. This is your weekly movement consistency day.

Today I would love you to do a movement practice you enjoy for about 45 minutes. You can go longer if you want, but choose something you can do consistently, easily. If you are already practising movement every day, try something new and be deliberate.

Go for a walk, take a yoga class, ride your bike, lift some weights, do some gardening, or do anything else you enjoy.

Completed! [   ]

Day 85. Practise and Share Gratitude

As we near the end of the 100-day challenge, it's helpful to think about how fortunate we are to have the life we have and how we can share this awareness with others in the hope that gratitude can make the world a better place.

To practise and share gratitude, I would love you to write a letter to a friend, FaceTime your family members or friends, or send a text to someone you care about and tell them why you appreciate them.

At work you can leave a sticky note on a co-worker's desk, thank them in an email, or tell them in person. These are simple ways to build gratitude and appreciate those in your life, the connections you have with them, and how they have helped you.

Make it a habit to thank at least one person every day.

Completed! [   ]

Day 86. Tum-Mo Breathing

Way back in chapter 1 (Breathe), I talked about tum-mo breathing, and you have already practised the breath of fire earlier in the 100-day challenge. Today we return to the practice so you can compare your mental strength to where you were earlier in the experience.

Tum-mo means heat. Research has demonstrated that trained Tibetan monks are able to raise the temperature of their fingers and toes during this practice by up to 7 °C. That is probably beyond us, but we can use tum-mo breathing to give us an energy boost.

Tum-mo breathing is a combination of two elements: a breathing pattern matched with a visualization. The visualization often involves imagining a flame moving up and down your spine.

Sit comfortably with good posture and take a few deep breaths.

Consciously relax your body and bring your attention to the here and now. Allow your mind to settle and quiet. Close your eyes.

Take a few moments to visualize a flame in the air just in front of your body. Now enclose that flame in a hollow balloon, with the ball of fire inside the balloon. Imagine bringing the fire inside your belly.

Keep this image active throughout the practice. When your mind wanders, gently bring your attention back to the fire.

Keep visualizing the internal fire, breathing smoothly and slowly as you feel the heat in your belly.

Gently extend the spine to look up as you inhale, and relax your spine back to a neutral position as you exhale.

Extend your spine tall and look slightly upward as you inhale, then relax your spine as you exhale so that your head returns to a neutral position.

Allow your chest to expand and shoulders to drop back as you inhale. As you exhale, allow your chest and ribs to relax, and bring your shoulders back to a neutral position.

Visualize the flame moving up your spine as you inhale, and down your spine as you exhale.

Try this for 10 slow inhale and exhale cycles.

Bring your attention back to your physical body and the environment around you. Open your eyes and enjoy the energy, heat, and mental activation.

Completed! [   ]

Day 87. Strengthen Your Muscles and Mitochondria
Back to resistance training today. Any of the following activities will get you your challenge point:

- Weight training
- Yoga
- Housework (vacuuming, cleaning, etc.)
- Gardening
- A spinning class
- Rowing
- Paddling
- Climbing
- Or any other type of exercise that strengthens your muscles

Completed! [   ]

Day 88. Today We Play

Let's have some fun today. All I want you to do is play. Here are a few ideas:

Colour. In the last decade, adult colouring books have become a trendy new form of creative play that is beneficial for many reasons. Colouring has even been suggested as an alternative form of meditation, as it allows us to switch our brains off and relax and focus on the task at hand, which reduces any pent-up tension, stress, and anxiety.

Try your hand at puzzles. Not only are puzzles a great way to wind down at the end of a long day and release built-up stress, but they also have incredible cognitive and mental health benefits. Some different puzzles you can try include crosswords, jigsaw puzzles, sudoku, dominos, checkers, and chess. For an even more immersive experience, try your hand at an escape room.

Play outdoor games. Exercise is perhaps the most important health-promoting practice and may also be one of the reasons why play is so healthy. Any form of play is great, so get out and play tennis or Frisbee, organize a soccer match, ride your bike, or fly a kite. The possibilities are endless.

Play with your pet. Have you ever heard of puppy therapy? It turns out that interacting with animals causes your body to produce the feel-good hormones serotonin and dopamine, which promote mental health and alleviate depression and anxiety. So take some time out of your day to pet your cat, or even better, take your play outside and go for a walk or play fetch with your dog.

Play with others. Group play also helps us build relationships and learn to work as a team. Some great collaborative ways that you can play with others include escape rooms, board games, and organized sports.

Completed! [   ]

Day 89. The Digital Pollution Detox

Part of maintaining our health, wellbeing, and mitochondrial energy is protecting our gains and ensuring that we continue to grow. I want to specifically ensure that your environment is set up for you to be successful after you are finished this 100-day challenge—which you have almost completed.

To that end, I respectfully suggest that you conduct a digital audit of all the media influences you have set up. Let's make sure you streamline your information and keep everything as positive as you can.

Here are some ideas for eliminating what I now refer to as digital pollution:

- Drop anyone you follow on social media who is in any way negative. If they don't elevate your life, unfollow and delete.
- Unsubscribe from any video platform subscriptions that are not informative and aligned with your dreams, goals, and ikigai.
- Unsubscribe from any podcasts or news sources that are not mission critical. I have one digital news subscription, and I subscribe to four podcasts. That's it.
- Unfollow any of your contacts on social media who are not positive influences on your life. You can still be friends, but you may not want to see their political posts.

Now that you have some space, you can curate your social media and news feed. Make everything that enters your brain worthy of your new levels of energy and attention.

Set a very high bar and protect it.

Completed! [   ]

Day 90. Live Slowly and Simply

Here are a few ideas for living simply and slowly that you can implement in your life to protect your new-found health, well-being, and energy.

Slow down. Meditation is a great way to slow down and appreciate the brevity of life. It allows us to ground ourselves in the present moment and focus our attention and awareness. The benefits of gratitude meditation, a positive psychological practice, overlap with those of both gratitude and meditative practices to promote overall health and wellbeing.* Take 10 minutes out of your day to follow along with a guided gratitude meditation video of your choice.

Live simply. Walk to the grocery store instead of taking your car, or turn off the air conditioning in your room for a few nights. The next time you indulge in these creature comforts, you'll appreciate them so much more. Live simply and you'll be that much more appreciative of the things you take for granted in your life.

Today just simplify your life or slow down deliberately for a few minutes to win today's challenge.

Completed! [   ]

Day 91. Your Movement Practice

Remember, the foundation of your mitochondrial challenge is consistent movement, and this is a practice. This is your weekly movement consistency day.

Today I would love you to do a movement practice you enjoy for about 45 minutes. You can go longer if you want, but choose something you can do consistently, easily. If you are already practising movement every day, try something new and be deliberate.

Go for a walk, take a yoga class, ride your bike, lift some weights, do some gardening, or do anything else you enjoy.

Completed! [   ]

---

* Selva, J. "Gratitude meditation: A simple but powerful happiness intervention." PositivePsychology.com (April 21, 2017). https://positivepsychology.com /gratitude-meditation-happiness.

Day 92. The Breath of Joy

Today is the last breathing day of the 100-day challenge, so let's do the breath of joy together.

Following this practice can release tensions and increase your natural life force, or "prana," thus both generating and opening yourself to receiving joy.

Here are the simple instructions:

1. Stand with your feet shoulder-width apart and arms at your sides.
2. Inhale to one-third of your lung capacity while you bring your arms up in front of your body to shoulder level, with palms facing each other.
3. Now inhale to two-thirds capacity and stretch your arms out to the sides, still at shoulder height.
4. Now inhale to full capacity and raise your arms over your head as if you're reaching for the sky.
5. Finally, exhale through your mouth as you lean forward and "take a bow," with your arms stretched out to the sides and slightly behind you. As you finish this motion and exhalation, smile and laugh.

Repeat this sequence four more times, for five times in total. As you become more familiar and comfortable with the combination of breathing and movements, try closing your eyes through each sequence and focusing your mind on the energy you feel circulating through your body.

Combining breathing with simple movements and a simple "clearing" visualization increases oxygen, decreases tension, improves mood and mental clarity, and invites more joy into your mind and body.

Completed! [   ]

Day 93. Do What You Love

The key to staying with an exercise program over time is quite simple. If you do activities you enjoy, you are more likely to do them more often. As I mentioned in chapter 2 (Move), female health care workers who experienced flow during a 12-week football (soccer) or Zumba intervention had greater adherence to physical activity 18 weeks later.

I love to paddleboard and swim. These are easy for me to motivate myself to do. So today just do an activity you enjoy that builds your physical health. Any form of exercise works.

Let's build the practices you will sustain once this challenge is over one week from now.

Completed! [   ]

Day 94. Overcome Your Cravings

Fasting has been a key practice for me over the last five years or so. I know it is very late in this challenge, but for the next few days I want to share ideas that will strengthen your mind–body connection so you are guaranteed success moving forward.

I would like you to consider, for the next week, adopting a 16:8 pattern for your nutrition. Eat within an eight-hour window and fast for 16 hours. If you want more information, check out power-up #1 in chapter 3 (Energize).

But here is the key that makes this challenge a bit different from just eating within a window of time. I want you to pay attention to when you get cravings for food or when you notice a drop in your energy levels. When you have a desire to eat, I want you to relax and breathe. Allow 5 to 10 minutes to pass. If after the 10 minutes you are still truly hungry, then by all means have a healthy snack or meal. However, I want you to practise your mental strength.

Be deliberate. Be healthy. Stay hydrated. Eat for healing and wellbeing. Let go of the patterns that no longer serve you. Set the stage for exponential energy.

If you manage to breathe through a craving or energy dip, you win today's challenge.

PS: If you have any history of disordered eating, you can skip this challenge today and go for a walk, read a book, or do any other practice you love to get your point.

Completed! [   ]

Day 95. Get Hot and Not Bothered

Let's do heat exposure one more time as we're finishing up the 100-day challenge.

Take a hot bath, have a sauna, or practise sunbathing in warm cor.di·· ıs.

· · your body respond and thrive. Notice your strength of ...ıd now compared with when you began this 100-day journey a few months ago.

Completed! [   ]

Day 96. Get Cool and Mindful

Just as we got hot yesterday, today we are cooling off.

Take a cold shower with the water cascading over your forehead and shoulders.

Or if you are ready, fill the bathtub with cold water from the tap and immerse your lower body for 5 to 10 minutes.

If you are feeling adventurous, then maybe take a dip in a cold lake or the ocean. As I write these words, I am mentally preparing for a cold plunge a few minutes from now.

While you are in the cold shower, bath, or body of water, bring your attention into the present moment and allow the discomfort of the cold water to simply pass you by.

Enjoy the health benefits and the mental concentration that comes with all your new experiences.

Completed! [   ]

Day 97. Enjoy a Healthy Meal

Today I encourage you to have a special meal with your family and loved ones.

Make something special. You can also order a healthy meal from your favourite restaurant.

Enjoy the organic proteins, the healthy fats, the colourful vegetables and fruits, and the spices and sauces.

Celebrate your success.

Completed! [   ]

Day 98. Your Movement Practice

This is your last movement practice for the challenge. Choose what you enjoy and get out there and go for it!

Please share your workout with me on social @drgregwells, and I will be sure to send you a note of congratulations. You are fantastic.

The VIIVIO app (download at www.viiv.io) helps you track your workouts, but it also gives you daily tips you can use to keep your learning going and to keep getting healthier and fitter after the challenge is finished. I also send out my podcast and newsletter via the app.

Completed! [   ]

Day 99. My Three Wins

You are on day 99 of a 100-day challenge. Congratulations! You have done brilliantly.

Remember that when we look back on our accomplishments and deliberately acknowledge and celebrate them, we build our confidence that we can continue to make progress and overcome any challenge we are faced with.

So today I would like you to look back over the 100-day challenge and give yourself credit for three things you added to your life that were positive. You only need to have tried three things and you win today's daily challenge.

My win #1:

My win #2:

My win #3:

Ping me with your awesomeness @drgregwells on Instagram or Twitter.

Completed! [   ]

Day 100. Start, Stop, Continue

Congratulations. You have reached the end of the challenge. You did awesome.

Let's again look back on what you've learned and think about what you want to do moving forward.

Are there certain ideas you tried that worked well for you? Are there some concepts you tried to implement but were not for you?

Today I'd like you to reflect on those ideas that worked and make a note so you can instill these practices in your life. Take a few minutes to ponder and answer these questions.

What practice(s) would you like to start?

What habit(s) would you like to stop?

What practice(s) do you want to continue?

Let me know what is working for you on Instagram or Twitter @drgregwells.

Completed! [   ]

The Final Word

You have done it and I am so proud of you. You are truly a gift to the world. I wish you all the best as you move forward with health, wellbeing, and new-found energy.

To keep the learning going, feel free to do any or all of the following:

1. Connect with me on Instagram or Twitter @drgregwells. I am honoured and grateful to connect with you.
2. Subscribe to my podcast: https://drgregwells.com/podcast.
3. Check out our YouTube channel: http://www.youtube.com/c /GregWellsPhD.
4. Visit my blog and you will be prompted to sign up for our news-letter: https://drgregwells.com/blog.
5. Download VIIVIO, our free health and wellbeing coaching app, at www.viiv.io.
6. Check out my previous books at https://drgregwells.com/books.

Yours in health and wellbeing,

Greg Wells, Ph.D.

ACKNOWLEDGEMENTS

Everything always begins and ends with my family. Judith, Ingrid, and Adam are wonderful and add magic to every single day of my life. They support and enable me to do everything that I do personally and professionally, including writing this book. I am deeply grateful to them for being awesome, for making my life incredible, and for their unwavering support.

For the last 20 years I have had the chance to do research at the Hospital for Sick Children in Toronto in the Translational Medicine program. My colleagues there have challenged me and helped me learn throughout those exciting and interesting decades. My grad students, including Dr. Sarah West, Dr. Gillian White, and Dr. Jessica Caterini, laid the groundwork for lines of research and thinking that have helped so many children with health challenges, and I am so honoured to have had them on my lab team. I am truly standing on the shoulders of so many giants in the scientific and research community whenever I write a book, and this book is no exception.

ACKNOWLEDGEMENTS

Over the last 10 years I've been building the Wells Performance consulting team. It has been an amazing project and I love knowledge translation, which is taking research and science and sharing it with the world in a way that's understandable and actionable. My team has been phenomenal and truly critical in the development of this book. Sara Thompson and Kate Rendall in particular did loads of research and background writing for many of the power-ups that appear in this book. I am so grateful to my incredible team, and I love spending my professional life with you all. Thanks so much.

One of the most fun things I do is interview spectacular humans for my podcast. I've referenced the learning and insights from these amazing humans who have appeared on the show in the power-ups and the words of wisdom that appear throughout this book. I am so grateful for my community and for the people who tune in every week to listen.

And finally, I'd like to thank my brilliant editor, Brad Wilson, and the entire HarperCollins publishing team. I am so grateful to have a publisher who holds me to the highest standards and takes my ideas and helps me share them with the world. I am so deeply grateful to have the opportunity to publish my fifth book with you.

NOTES

Introduction: An Upward Spiral of Wellness

1. "The origin of mitochondria and chloroplasts." Nature Education (2014). https://www.nature.com/scitable/content/the-origin-of-mitochondria-and-chloroplasts-14747702.

2. Sneed, A. "The origin of power." *Scientific American* 312, no. 2 (February 2015): 20–21.

3. "What are mitochondria and why they matter." MitoCanada (2022). https://mitocanada.org/understanding-mito/what-are-mitochondria.

4. MitoCanada. "What are mitochondria?"

5. Pizzorno, J. "Mitochondria—fundamental to life and health." *Integrative Medicine* (Encinitas) 13, no. 2 (April 2014): 8–15.

6. Javadov, S., A.V. Kozlov, and A.K.S. Camara. "Mitochondria in health and diseases." *Cells* 9, no. 5 (May 9, 2020): 1177.

7. Haas, R. "Mitochondrial dysfunction in aging and diseases of aging." *Biology* (Basel, CH) 8, no. 2 (2019): 48.

8. Pizzorno. "Mitochondria."

9. Panchal, N., R. Kamal, C. Cox, and R. Garfield. "The implications of COVID-19 for mental health and substance use." Kaiser Family Foundation (February 10, 2021).

10. Pizzorno. "Mitochondria."

11. Tsiloulis, T., and M.J. Watt. "Exercise and the regulation of adipose tissue metabolism." In *Progress in Molecular Biology and Translational Science*, vol. 135, ed. L. Zhang, 175–201 (Cambridge, MA: Academic Press, 2015).

Chapter 1: Breathe

1. Wells, G.D., M. Plyley, S. Thomas, L. Goodman, and J. Duffin. "Effects of concurrent inspiratory and expiratory muscle training on respiratory and exercise performance in competitive swimmers." *European Journal of Applied Physiology* 94, no. 5–6 (August 2005): 527–540.

2. Tsiloulis, T., and M.J. Watt. "Exercise and the regulation of adipose tissue metabolism." In *Progress in Molecular Biology and Translational Science*, vol. 135, ed. L. Zhang, 175–201 (Cambridge, MA: Academic Press, 2015).

3. King, A. "Could mitochondria help athletes to make gains? The muscles of elite endurance athletes boast high numbers of extra-efficient mitochondria. Unlocking the secrets of these cellular components could yield gains for future Olympians." *Nature* 592 (March 31, 2021): S7–S9.

4. Benson, H., R.F. Steinert, M.M. Greenwood, H.M. Klemchuk, and N.H. Peterson. "Continuous measurement of O_2 consumption and CO_2 elimination during a wakeful hypometabolic state." *Journal of Human Stress* 1, no. 1 (1975): 37–44.

5. Dempsey, J. "The biomedical basis of elite performance." Paper presented at the Physiological Society conference, Madison, Wisconsin (March 19–21, 2012). YouTube video 45:29. https://www.youtube.com/watch?v=92NRGg9vjD4.

6. Gimenez-Palomo, A., S. Dodd, G. Anmella, A.F. Carvalho, G. Scaini, J. Quevedo, I. Pacchiarotti, E. Vieta, and M. Berk. "The role of mitochondria in mood disorders: From physiology to pathophysiology and to treatment." *Frontiers in Psychiatry* (July 6, 2021).

7. In an article for the *Journal of Young Investigators*, Shilpa Gowda makes a case: Gowda, S. "New insight into panic attacks: Carbon dioxide is the culprit." *Journal of Young Investigators* (November 10, 2007).

8. Benson, H., J.F. Beary, and M.P. Carol. "The relaxation response." *Psychiatry* 37, no. 1 (1974): 37–46.

9. Zaccaro A., A. Piarulli, M. Laurino, E. Garbella, D. Menicucci, B. Neri, and A. Gemignani. "How breath-control can change your life: A systematic review on psycho-physiological correlates of slow breathing." *Frontiers in Human Neuroscience* 12 (September 7, 2018): 353.

10. "Global prevalence and burden of depressive and anxiety disorders in 204 countries and territories in 2020 due to the COVID-19 pandemic." *The Lancet* 398, no. 10312 (November 6, 2021): P1700–P1712.

11. American Psychological Association. *Stress in America 2020: A National Mental Health Crisis* (Washington: APA, 2020).

12. The Data Team. "How heavy use of social media is linked to mental illness." *The Economist* (updated December 7, 2018). https://www.economist.com/graphic-detail/2018/05/18/how-heavy-use-of-social-media-is-linked-to-mental-illness.

13. The Data Team. "Generation Z is stressed, depressed and exam-obsessed." *The Economist* (February 27, 2019). https://www.economist.com/graphic-detail/2019/02/27/generation-z-is-stressed-depressed-and-exam-obsessed.

14. Landau, E. "Mitochondria may hold keys to anxiety and mental health." *Quanta Magazine* (August 10, 2020). https://www.quantamagazine.org/mitochondria-may-hold-keys-to-anxiety-and-mental-health-20200810.

15. Landau. "Mitochondria may hold keys."

16. Rezin, G.T., G. Amboni, A.I. Zugno, J. Quevedo, and E.L. Streck. "Mitochondrial dysfunction and psychiatric disorders." *Neurochemistry Research* 34, no. 6 (June 2009): 1021–1029.

17. Picard, M., and B.S. McEwen. "Psychological stress and mitochondria: A systematic review." *Psychosomatic Medicine* 80, no. 2 (February/March 2018): 141–153.

18. Dusek, J.A., H.H. Otu, A.L. Wohlhueter, M. Bhasin, L.F. Zerbini, M.G. Joseph, H. Benson, and T.A. Libermann. "Genomic counter-stress changes induced by the relaxation response." *PLoS One* 3, no. 7 (July 2, 2008): e2576.

19. Zaccaro et al. "Breath-control can change your life."

20. Alderman, L. "Breathe. Exhale. Repeat: The benefits of controlled breathing." *New York Times* (November 9, 2016).

21. Yackle, K., L.A. Schwarz, K. Kam, J.M. Sorokin, J.R. Huguenard, J.L. Feldman, L. Luo, and M.A. Krasnow. "Breathing control center neurons that promote arousal in mice." *Science* 355 no. 6332 (March 31, 2017): 1411–1415.

22. Siegel, R.D., C.K. Germer, and A. Olendzki. "Mindfulness: What is it? Where did it come from?" In *Clinical Handbook of Mindfulness*, ed. F. Didonna, 17–35 (New York: Springer, 2009).

23. McClintock, A.S., S.M. McCarrick, E.L. Garland, F. Zeidan, and A.E. Zgierska. "Brief mindfulness-based interventions for acute and chronic pain: A systematic review." *Journal of Alternate Complementary Medicine* 25, no. 3 (March 2019): 265–278.

24. Kabat-Zinn, J. "An outpatient program in behavioral medicine for chronic pain patients based on the practice of mindfulness meditation: Theoretical considerations and preliminary results." *General Hospital Psychiatry* 4, no. 1 (April 1982): 33–47.

25. Schuman-Olivier, Z., M. Trombka, D.A. Lovas, J.A. Brewer, D.R. Vago, R. Gawande, J.P. Dunne, S.W. Lazar, E.B. Loucks, and C. Fulwiler. "Mindfulness and behavior change." *Harvard Review of Psychiatry* 28, no. 6 (November/December 2020): 371–394.

26. Wells, R.E., E.K. Seng, R.R. Edwards, D.E. Victorson, C.R. Pierce, L. Rosenberg, V. Napadow, and Z. Schuman-Olivier. "Mindfulness in migraine: A narrative review." *Expert Review of Neurotherapeutics* 20, no. 3 (March 2020): 207–225.

27. Yusufov, M., J. Nicoloro-Santa Barbara, N.E. Grey, A. Moyer, and M. Lobel. "Meta-analytic evaluation of stress reduction interventions for undergraduate and graduate students." *International Journal of Stress Management* 26, no. 2 (2019): 132–145.

28. Baer, R.A. "Mindfulness training as a clinical intervention: A conceptual and empirical review." *Clinical Psychology: Science and Practice* 10, no. 2 (2003): 125–143.

29. Bishop, S.R., M. Lau, S. Shapiro, L.E. Carlson, N.D. Anderson, J. Carmody, Z.V. Segal, S. Abbey, M. Speca, D. Velting, and G. Devins. "Mindfulness: A proposed operational definition." *Clinical Psychology Science and Practice* 11 (2004): 230–241.

30. Shapiro, S.L., L.E. Carlson, J.A. Astin, and B. Freedman. "Mechanisms of mindfulness." *Journal of Clinical Psychology* 62, no. 3 (March 2006): 373–386.

31. Mumford, G. *The Mindful Athlete: Secrets to Pure Performance* (Berkeley, CA: Parallax Press, 2015).

32. "Mindful breathing: A way to build resilience to stress, anxiety, and anger." Greater Good in Action. [Accessed October 6, 2022.] https://ggia.berkeley.edu/practice/mindful_breathing.

33. Vago, D.R., and D.A. Silbersweig. "Self-awareness, self-regulation, and self-transcendence (S-ART): A framework for understanding the neurobiological mechanisms of mindfulness." *Frontiers in Human Neuroscience* 25, no. 6 (October 2012): 296.

34. Roy, A., S. Druker, E.A. Hoge, and J.A. Brewer. "Physician anxiety and burnout: Symptom correlates and a prospective pilot study of app-delivered mindfulness training." *JMIR mHealth and uHealth* 8, no. 4 (April 1, 2020): e15608.

35. Gerritsen, R.J.S., and G.P.H. Band. "Breath of life: The respiratory vagal stimulation model of contemplative activity." *Frontiers in Human Neuroscience* 12 (October 9, 2018): 397.

36. Geisler, F.C.M., M.N. Bechtoldt, N. Oberländer, and M. Schacht-Jablonowsky. "The benefits of a mindfulness exercise in a performance situation." *Psychological Reports* 121, no. 5 (October 2018): 853–876.

37. Trinity College Dublin. "The Yogi masters were right—meditation and breathing exercises can sharpen your mind." ScienceDaily (May 10, 2018). www.sciencedaily.com/releases/2018/05/180510101254.htm.

38. Melnychuk, M.C., P.M. Dockree, G. Redmond, P.R. O'Connell, J.H. Murphy, J.H. Balsters, and I.H. Robertson. "Coupling of respiration and attention via the locus coeruleus: Effects of meditation and pranayama." *Psychophysiology* (April 22, 2018): e13091.

39. Fumoto, M., I. Sato-Suzuki, Y. Seki, Y. Mohri, and H. Arita. "Appearance of high-frequency alpha band with disappearance of low-frequency alpha band in EEG is produced during voluntary abdominal breathing in an eyes-closed condition." *Neuroscience Research* 50, no. 3 (November 2004): 307–317.

40. Telles, S., R. Nagarathna, and H.R. Nagendra. "Breathing through a particular nostril can alter metabolism and autonomic activities." *Indian Journal of Physiology and Pharmacology* 38, no. 2 (April 1994): 133–137.

41. Kamath, A., R.P. Urval, and A.K. Shenoy. "Effect of alternate nostril breathing exercise on experimentally induced anxiety in healthy volunteers using the simulated public speaking model: A randomized controlled pilot study." *Biomed Research International* 2017 (2017): 2450670.

42. Zelano, C., H. Jiang, G. Zhou, N. Arora, S. Schuele, J. Rosenow, and J.A. Gottfried. "Nasal respiration entrains human limbic oscillations and modulates cognitive function." *Journal of Neuroscience* 36, no. 49 (December 7, 2016): 12448–12467.

43. Bongers, C.C.W.G., T.M.H. Eijsvogels, D.H.J. Thijssen, and M.T.E. Hopman. "Thermoregulatory, metabolic, and cardiovascular responses during 88 min of full-body ice immersion—a case study." *Physiological Reports* 7, no. 24 (December 2019): e14304.

44. Benson, H., J. Lehmann, M. Malhotra, R. Goldman, J. Hopkins, and M.D. Epstein. "Body temperature changes during the practice of tum-mo yoga." *Nature* 295 (1982): 234–236.

45. Newman, R.W. "Temperature regulation training in a cooling environment." *American Industrial Hygiene Association Journal* (June 4, 2010): 610–617.

46. Cromie, W.J. "Meditation changes temperatures: Mind controls body in extreme experiments." *Harvard Gazette* (April 18, 2002).

47. Kozhevnikov, M., J. Elliott, J. Shephard, and K. Gramann. "Neurocognitive and somatic components of temperature increase during g-tummo meditation: Legend and reality." *PLoS One* 8, no. 3 (2013): e58244.

48. Andrew Hamilton makes a case: Hamilton, A. "Respiratory training: Why your breathing muscles matter for endurance." *Sports Performance Bulletin* (2022).

49. Mortola, J.P. "How to breathe? Respiratory mechanics and breathing pattern." *Respiratory Physiology and Neurobiology* 261 (March 2019): 48–54.

50. Hinterberger, T., N. Walter, C. Doliwa, and T. Loew. "The brain's resonance with breathing-decelerated breathing synchronizes heart rate and slow cortical potentials." *Journal of Breath Research* 13, no. 4 (June 27, 2019): 046003.

51. Wagner G.D. "3 exercises to increase your lung power." *Active* (June 26, 2018).

52. Gerritsen and Band. "Breath of life."

53. Johnson, M.K. "Joy: A review of the literature and suggestions for future directions." *Journal of Positive Psychology* 15, no. 1 (November 19, 2019).

54. Zope, S.A., and R.A. Zope. "Sudarshan Kriya yoga: Breathing for health." *International Journal of Yoga* 6, no. 1 (January 2013): 4–10.

55. Zope and Zope. "Sudarshan Kriya yoga."

Chapter 2: Move

1. Wilkes, D.L., J.E. Schneiderman, T. Nguyen, L. Heale, F. Moola, F. Ratjen, A.L. Coates, and G.D. Wells. "Exercise and physical activity in children with cystic fibrosis." *Paediatric Respiratory Reviews* 10, no. 3 (September 2009): 105–109.

2. Memme, J.M., A.T. Erlich, G. Phukan, and D.A. Hood. "Exercise and mitochondrial health." Presented at the 2018 ACSM Integrative Physiology of Exercise conference, San Diego, California (September 5–8, 2018). https://doi.org/10.1113/JP278853.

3. King, A. "Could mitochondria help athletes to make gains? The muscles of elite endurance athletes boast high numbers of extra-efficient mitochondria. Unlocking the secrets of these cellular components could yield gains for future Olympians." *Nature* 592 (March 31, 2021): S7–S9.

4. Cogliati, S., C. Frezza, M.E. Soriano, T. Varanita, R. Quintana-Cabrera, M. Corrado, S. Cipolat, et al. "Mitochondrial cristae shape determines respiratory chain supercomplexes assembly and respiratory efficiency." *Cell* 155, no. 1 (September 26, 2013): 160–171.

5. Nielsen, J., K.D. Gejl, M. Hey-Mogensen, H.C. Holmberg, C. Suetta, P. Krustrup, C.P.H. Elemans, and N. Ørtenblad. "Plasticity in mitochondrial cristae density allows metabolic capacity modulation in human skeletal muscle." *Journal of Physiology* 595, no. 9 (May 1, 2017): 2839–2847.

6. Huertas, J.R., R.A. Casuso, P.H. Agustin, and S. Cogliati. "Stay fit, stay young: Mitochondria in movement: The role of exercise in the new mitochondrial paradigm." *Oxidative Medicine and Cellular Longevity* 2019 (June 19, 2019).

7. Greggio, C., P. Jha, S.S. Kulkarni, S. Lagarrigue, N.T. Broskey, M. Boutant, X. Wang, et al. "Enhanced respiratory chain supercomplex formation in response to exercise in human skeletal muscle." *Cell Metabolism* 25, no. 2 (February 7, 2017): 301–311.

8. Adães, S. "Why does mitochondrial health affect aging? 4 science-backed ways to rejuvenate mitochondria." *Neurohacker Collective* (June 14, 2021). https://neurohacker.com/why-does-mitochondrial-health-affect-aging-4-science-backed-ways-to-rejuvenate-mitochondria.

9. Lundby, C., and R.A. Jacobs. "Movement is perhaps the most powerful stimulus to build and strengthen our mitochondria." *Experimental Physiology* 101, no. 1 (January 1, 2016): 17–22.

10. Menshikova, E.V., V.B. Ritov, L. Fairfull, R.E. Ferrell, D.E. Kelley, and B.H. Goodpaster. "Effects of exercise on mitochondrial content and function in aging human skeletal muscle." *Journals of Gerontology Series A Biological Sciences and Medical Sciences* 61, no. 6 (June 2006): 534–640.

11. Paluch, A.E., K.P. Gabriel, J.E. Fulton, C.E. Lewis, P.J. Schreiner, B. Sternfeld, S. Sidney, et al. "Steps per day and all-cause mortality in middle-aged adults in the Coronary Artery Risk Development in Young Adults study." *JAMA Network Open* 4, no. 9 (September 3, 2021): e2124516.

12. Schnohr, P., J.H. O'Keefe, C.J. Lavie, A. Holtermann, P. Lange, G.B. Jensen, and J.L. Marott. "U-shaped association between duration of sports activities and mortality: Copenhagen City Heart Study." *Mayo Clinic Proceedings* 96, no. 12 (August 17, 2021): 3012–3020. www.mayoclinicproceedings.org/article/S0025-6196(21)00475-4/fulltext.

13. Ekelund, U., J. Tarp, M.W. Fagerland, J.S. Johannessen, B.H. Hansen, B.J. Jefferis, P.H. Whincup, et al. "Joint associations of accelerometer-measured physical activity and sedentary time with all-cause mortality: A harmonised meta-analysis in more than 44,000 middle-aged and older individuals." *British Journal of Sports Medicine* 54, no. 24 (December 2020): 1499–1506.

14. Jacobs, R.A., and C. Lundby. "Mitochondria express enhanced quality as well as quantity in association with aerobic fitness across recreationally active individuals up to elite athletes." *Journal of Applied Physiology* (1985) 114, no. 3 (February 2013): 344–350.

15. Puntschart, A., H. Claassen, K. Jostarndt, H. Hoppeler, and R. Billeter. "mRNAs of enzymes involved in energy metabolism and mtDNA are increased in endurance-trained athletes." *American Journal of Physiology* 269, no. 3, pt. 1 (September 1995): C619–C625.

16. Starritt, E.C., D. Angus, and M. Hargreaves. "Effect of short-term training on mitochondrial ATP production rate in human skeletal muscle." (February 1, 1999). https://journals.physiology.org/doi/full/10.1152/jappl.1999.86.2.450.

17. Pedersen, B.K., and B. Saltin. "Exercise as medicine—evidence for prescribing exercise as therapy in 26 different chronic diseases." *Scandinavian Journal of Medicine and Science in Sports* (November 25, 2015). https://onlinelibrary.wiley.com/doi/10.1111/sms.12581.

18. Park, J.H., J.H. Moon, H.J. Kim, M.H. Kong, and Y.H. Oh. "Sedentary lifestyle: Overview of updated evidence of potential health risks." *Korean Journal of Family Medicine* 41, no. 6 (November 2020): 365–373.

19. Oppezzo, M., and D.L. Schwartz. "Give your ideas some legs: The positive effect of walking on creative thinking." *Journal of Experimental Psychology: Learning, Memory, and Cognition* 40, no. 4 (2014): 1142–1152. www.apa.org/pubs/journals/releases/xlm-a0036577.pdf.

20. Colmenares, A.M., M.W. Voss, J. Fanning, E.A. Salerno, N.P. Gothe, M.L. Thomas, E. McCauley, A.F. Kramer, and A.Z. Burzynska. "White matter plasticity in healthy older adults: The effects of aerobic exercise." *NeuroImage* 1, no. 239 (October 2021): 118305.

21. Yates, T., M. Davies, E. Brady, D. Webb, T. Gorely, F. Bull, D. Talbot, N. Sattar, and K. Khunti. "Walking and inflammatory markers in individuals screened for type 2 diabetes." *Preventive Medicine* 47, no. 4 (October 2008): 417–421.

22. Hori, H., A. Ikenouchi-Sugita, R. Yoshimura, and J. Nakamura. "Does subjective sleep quality improve by a walking intervention? A real-world study in a Japanese workplace." *BMJ Open* 6, no. 10 (October 24, 2016): e011055.

23. Fiorenzi, R. "Sitting is the new smoking." Start Standing (May 15, 2022). www.startstanding.org/sitting-new-smoking/#para1.

24. "An 'awe walk' might do wonders for your well-being." *New York Times* (September 30, 2020). www.nytimes.com/2020/09/30/well /move/an-awe-walk-might-do-wonders-for-your-well-being.html.

25. van Dam, K. "Individual stress prevention through qigong." *International Journal of Environmental Research and Public Health* 17, no. 19 (October 2020): 7342. https://www.mdpi.com/1660-4601/17/19/7342.

26. Mindful staff. "What is mindfulness? Are you supposed to clear your mind, or focus on one thing? Here's the Mindful definition of mindfulness." Mindful (July 8, 2020). www.mindful.org/what-is-mindfulness.

27. Mayo Clinic staff. "Mindfulness exercises: See how mindfulness helps you live in the moment." Healthy Lifestyle: Consumer Health. Mayo Clinic (September 15, 2020). www.mayoclinic.org/healthy-lifestyle /consumer-health/in-depth/mindfulness-exercises/art-20046356.

28. Wang, F., and A. Szabo. "Effects of yoga on stress among healthy adults: A systematic review." *Alternative Therapies in Health and Medicine* 26, no. 4 (July 2020): AT6214.

29. Goldstein, M.R., R.K. Lewin, and J.J.B. Allen. "Improvements in well-being and cardiac metrics of stress following a yogic breathing workshop: Randomized controlled trial with active comparison." *Journal of American College Health* 70, no. 3 (2022): 918–928.

30. Nguyen, M.H., and A. Kruse. "A randomized controlled trial of tai chi for balance, sleep quality and cognitive performance in elderly Vietnamese." *Clinical Interventions in Aging* 7 (2012): 185–190.

31. Solianik, R., D. Mickevičienė, L. Žlibinaitė, and A. Čekanauskaitė. "Tai chi improves psychoemotional state, cognition, and motor learning in older adults during the COVID-19 pandemic." *Experimental Gerontology* 150 (July 15, 2021): 111363.

32. Huston, P., and B. McFarlane. "Health benefits of tai chi. What is the

evidence?" *Canadian Family Physician* 62, no. 11 (November 2016): 881–890.

33. Ho, R.T., C.W. Wang, S.M. Ng, A.H. Ho, E.T. Ziea, V.T. Wong, and C.L. Chan. "The effect of t'ai chi exercise on immunity and infections: A systematic review of controlled trials." *Journal of Alternative and Complementary Medicine* (New York) 19, no. 5 (May 2013): 389–396.

34. van Dam. "Individual stress prevention through qigong."

35. Gerritsen, R.J.S., and G.P.H. Band. "Breath of life: The respiratory vagal stimulation model of contemplative activity." *Frontiers in Human Neuroscience* 9, no. 12 (October 2018): 397.

36. "Exercise can boost your memory and thinking skills." Mind & Mood. Harvard Health Publishing (February 15, 2021). www.health.harvard.edu/mind-and-mood/exercise-can-boost-your-memory-and-thinking-skills.

37. Torma, F., Z. Gombos, M. Jokai, M. Takeda, T. Mimura, and Z. Radak. "High intensity interval training and molecular adaptive response of skeletal muscle." *Sports Medicine and Health Science* 1, no. 1 (December 2019): 24–32.

38. Robinson M.M, S. Dasari, A.R. Konopka, M.L. Johnson, S. Manjunatha, R.R. Esponda, R.E. Carter, I.R. Lanza, K.S. Nair. "Enhanced protein translation underlies improved metabolic and physical adaptations to different exercise training modes in young and old humans." *Cellular Metabolism* 25, no. 3 (March 7, 2017): 581–592.

39. Torma et al. "High intensity interval training."

40. Little, J.P., A. Safdar, D. Bishop, M.A. Tarnopolsky, and M.J. Gibala. "An acute bout of high-intensity interval training increases the nuclear abundance of PGC-1α and activates mitochondrial biogenesis in human skeletal muscle." *American Journal of Physiology: Regulatory, Integrative and Comparative Physiology* 300, no. 6 (June 1, 2011): R1303–R1310.

41. Walsh, J.J., and M.E. Tschakovsky. "Exercise and circulating BDNF: Mechanisms of release and implications for the design of exercise interventions." *Applied Physiology, Nutrition, and Metabolism* 43, no. 11 (November 2018): 1095–1104.

42. Little, J.P., J. Langley, M. Lee, E. Myette-Côté, G. Jackson, C. Durrer, M.J. Gibala, and M.E. Jung. "Sprint exercise snacks: A novel approach to increase aerobic fitness." *European Journal of Applied Physiology* 119 no. 5 (May 2019): 1203–1212.

43. Peifer, C., G. Wolters, L. Harmat, J. Heutte, J. Tan, T. Freire, D. Tavares, et al. "A scoping review of flow research." *Frontiers in Psychology* 2022, no. 13 (April 7, 2022): 815665.

44. Holt-Lunstad, J., T.B. Smith, and J.B. Layton. "Social relationships and mortality risk: A meta-analytic review." *PLoS Medicine* 7, no. 7 (July 27, 2010): e1000316.

45. Vance, E. "Channel all that rage into your workout." *New York Times* (August 11, 2021). https://www.nytimes.com/2021/08/11/well/move/workout-stress-fear.html.

46. Vance. "Channel all that rage."

47. Maestroni, L., P. Read, C. Bishop, K. Papadopoulos, T.J. Suchomel, P. Comfort, and A. Turner. "The benefits of strength training on musculoskeletal system health: Practical applications for interdisciplinary care." *Sports Medicine* (Auckland, NZ) 50, no. 8 (August 2020): 1431–1450.

48. Saeidifard, F., J.R. Medina-Inojosa, C.P. West, T.P. Olson, V.K. Somers, A.R. Bonikowske, L.J. Prokop, M. Vinciguerra, and F. Lopez-Jimenez. "The association of resistance training with mortality: A systematic review and meta-analysis." *European Journal of Preventive Cardiology* 26, no. 15 (October 2019): 1647–1665.

49. Porter, C., P.T. Reidy, N. Bhattarai, L.S. Sidossis, and B.B. Rasmussen. "Resistance exercise training alters mitochondrial function in human skeletal muscle." *Medicine & Science in Sports & Exercise* 47, no. 9 (September 2015): 1922–1931.

50. Pesta, D., F. Hoppel, C. Macek, H. Messner, M. Faulhaber, C. Kobel, W. Parson, M. Burtscher, M. Schocke, and E. Gnaiger. "Similar qualitative and quantitative changes of mitochondrial respiration following strength and endurance training in normoxia and hypoxiain sedentary humans." *American Journal of Physiology: Regulatory Integrated Comparative Physiology* 301 (October 2011): R1078–R1087.

51. Zeng, Z., J. Liang, L. Wu, H. Zhang, J. Lv, and N. Chen. "Exercise-induced autophagy suppresses sarcopenia through Akt/mTOR and

Akt/FoxO3a signal pathways and AMPK-mediated mitochondrial quality control." *Frontiers in Physiology* 2, no. 11 (November 2020): 583478.

52. Watson, K., and K. Baar. "mTOR and the health benefits of exercise." *Seminars in Cell & Developmental Biology* 36 (December 2014): 130–139.

53. Laplante, M., and D.M. Sabatin. "mTOR signaling in growth control and disease." *Cell* 149, no. 2 (April 13, 2012): 274–293.

54. Csikszentmihalyi, M. "FLOW: The psychology of optimal experience." Global Learning Communities (2000). https://mktgsensei .com/AMAE/Consumer%20Behavior/flow_the_psychology_of _optimal_experience.pdf.

55. Boudreau, P., S.H. Mackenzie, and K. Hodge. "Optimal psychological states in advanced climbers: Antecedents, characteristics, and consequences of flow and clutch states." *Psychology of Sport and Exercise* 60 (May 2022): 102155.

56. Jackson, S., and R.C. Eckland. *The Flow Scale Manual* (Morgantown: West Virginia University Press, 2004).

57. Elbe, A.M., S. Barene, K. Strahler, P. Krustrup, and A. Holtermann. "Experiencing flow in a workplace physical activity intervention for female health care workers: A longitudinal comparison between football and Zumba." *Women in Sport and Physical Activity Journal* 24, no. 1 (May 2016): 70–77. www.researchgate.net/publication/301799915.

58. Gold, J., and J. Ciorciari. "A review on the role of the neuroscience of flow states in the modern world." *Behavioral Sciences* (Basel, CH) 10, no. 9 (September 2020): 137.

59. Boudreau, Mackenzie, and Hodge. "Optimal psychological states in advanced climbers."

60. Health Canada. "Ventilation and the indoor environment." Government of Canada: Publications: Healthy Living (March 2018). www .canada.ca/en/health-canada/services/publications/healthy-living /ventilation-indoor-environment.html.

61. Gladwell, V.F., D.K. Brown, C. Wood, R.G. Sandercock, and J.L. Barton. "The great outdoors: How a green exercise environment can benefit all." *Extreme Physiology & Medicine* 2, no. 3 (2013). https://doi .org/10.1186/2046-7648-2-3.

62. Li, Q., T. Otsuka, M. Kobayashi, Y. Wakayama, H. Inagaki, M.Y. Katsumata, Y. Hirata, et al. "Acute effects of walking in forest environments on cardiovascular and metabolic parameters." *European Journal of Applied Physiology* 111, no. 11 (November 1, 2011): 2845–2853.

63. Olafsdottir, G., P. Cloke, A. Schulz, Z. van Dyck, T. Eysteinsson, B. Thorleifsdottir, and C. Vögele. "Health benefits of walking in nature: A randomized controlled study under conditions of real-life stress." *Environment and Behavior* 52, no. 3 (September 28, 2018). https://doi.org/10.1177/0013916518800798.

64. Ulrich, R.S., R.F. Simons, B.D. Losito, E. Fiorito, M.A. Miles, and M. Zelson. "Stress recovery during exposure to natural and urban environments." *Journal of Environmental Psychology* 11, no. 3 (September 11, 1991): 201–230.

65. Kotera, Y., M. Richardson, and D. Sheffield. "Effects of shinrin-yoku (forest bathing) and nature therapy on mental health: A systematic review and meta-analysis." *International Journal of Mental Health and Addiction* 20, no. 1 (February 1, 2022): 337–361.

66. Gladwell et al. "The great outdoors."

67. Lee, J., Y. Tsunetsugu, N. Takayama, B.J. Park, Q. Li, C. Song, M. Komatsu, et al. "Influence of forest therapy on cardiovascular relaxation in young adults." *Evidence-Based Complementary Alternative Medicine* 2014 (February 10, 2014): 834360.

68. Wood, C.J., J. Pretty, and M. Griffin. "A case-control study of the health and well-being benefits of allotment gardening." *Journal of Public Health* (Oxford, UK) 38, no. 3 (September 2016): e336–e344.

69. Focht, B.C. "Brief walks in outdoor and laboratory environments: Effects on affective responses, enjoyment, and intentions to walk for exercise." *Research Quarterly for Exercise and Sport* 80, no. 3 (September 2009): 611–620.

70. McDougall, C.W., R. Foley, N. Hanley, R.S. Quilliam, and D.M. Oliver. "Freshwater wild swimming, health and well-being: Understanding the importance of place and risk." *Sustainability* 14, no. 10 (January 2022): 6364.

71. van Tulleken, C., M. Tipton, H. Massey, and C.M. Harper. "Open water swimming as a treatment for major depressive disorder." *BMJ Case Reports* 2018 (August 21, 2018): bcr2018225007.

72. Ekkekakis, P., and R. Brand. "Affective responses to and automatic affective valuations of physical activity: Fifty years of progress on the seminal question in exercise psychology." *Psychology of Sport and Exercise* 42 (May 2019): 130–137.

73. van Geest, J., R. Samaritter, and S. van Hooren. "Move and be moved: The effect of moving specific movement elements on the experience of happiness." *Frontiers in Psychology* 11 (January 15, 2021). www .frontiersin.org/articles/10.3389/fpsyg.2020.579518/full.

74. Melzer, A., T. Shafir, and R.P. Tsachor. "How do we recognize emotion from movement? Specific motor components contribute to the recognition of each emotion." *Frontiers in Psychology* (July 3, 2019). https://doi.org/10.3389/fpsyg.2019.01389.

75. McGonigal, K. "The Joy Workout." Move. *New York Times* (May 24, 2022). www.nytimes.com/2022/05/24/well/move/joy-workout-exercises-happiness.html.

76. Reis, H.T., S.D. O'Keefe, and R.D. Lane. "Fun is more fun when others are involved." *Journal of Positive Psychology* 12, no. 6 (2017): 547–557.

77. van Geest, Samaritter, and van Hooren. "Move and be moved."

78. WHO Newsroom. "Physical activity." World Health Organization (June 15, 2022). www.who.int/news-room/fact-sheets/detail /physical-activity.

79. Little et al. "Sprint exercise snacks."

Chapter 3: Energize

1. Ricci, J.A., E. Chee, A.L. Lorandeau, and J. Berger. "Fatigue in the U.S. workforce: Prevalence and implications for lost productive work time." *Journal of Occupational and Environmental Medicine* 49, no. 1 (January 2007): 1–10.

2. Toppinen-Tanner, S., A. Ojajärvi, A. Väänänen, R. Kalimo, and P. Jäppinen. "Burnout as a predictor of medically certified sick-leave absences and their diagnosed causes." *Behavioral Medicine* (Washington, DC) 31, no. 1 (Spring 2005): 18–27.

3. Deligkaris, P., E. Panagopoulou, A.J. Montgomery, and E. Masoura. "Job burnout and cognitive functioning: A systematic review." *Work & Stress: An International Journal of Work, Health & Organisations* 28, no. 2 (April 30, 2014): 107–123.

4. Toppinen-Tanner et al. "Burnout as a predictor of medically certified sick-leave."

5. Zhang H., J. Wang, X. Geng, C. Li, and S. Wang. "Objective assessments of mental fatigue during a continuous long-term stress condition." *Frontiers of Human Neuroscience* (November 10, 2021): 15.

6. Van Cutsem, J., S. Marcora, K. De Pauw, S. Bailey, R. Meeusen, and B. Roelands. "The effects of mental fatigue on physical performance: A systematic review." *Sports Medicine* (Auckland, NZ) 47, no. 8 (August 2017): 1569–1588.

7. Calabrese, E.J., and W.J. Kozumbo. "The hormetic dose-response mechanism: Nrf2 activation." *Pharmacological Research* 167 (May 1, 2021): 105526.

8. Rossnerova, A., A. Izzotti, A. Pulliero, A. Bast, S.I.S. Rattan, and P. Rossner. "The molecular mechanisms of adaptive response related to environmental stress." *International Journal of Molecular Sciences* 21, no. 19 (September 25, 2020): 7053.

9. Ristow, M., and K. Schmeisser. "Mitohormesis: Promoting health and lifespan by increased levels of reactive oxygen species (ROS)." *Dose-Response* 12, no. 2 (January 31, 2014): 288–341.

10. Casado, Á., A. Castellanos, M.E. López-Fernández, R. Ruíz, C. García Aroca, and F. Noriega. "Relationship between oxidative and occupational stress and aging in nurses of an intensive care unit." *Age* (Dordrecht, NL) 30, no. 4 (December 2008): 229–236.

11. Held, P. "An introduction to reactive oxygen species measurement of ROS in cells." Semantic Scholar (2010). www.semanticscholar.org /paper/An-Introduction-to-Reactive-Oxygen-Species-of-ROS-Held /ed3385e1ac7f8d604e2d3e4fa91c668d925f51fe.

12. Santos, J.H., L. Hunakova, Y. Chen, C. Bortner, and B.V. Houten. "Cell sorting experiments link persistent mitochondrial DNA damage with loss of mitochondrial membrane potential and apoptotic cell death." *Journal of Biological Chemistry* 278, no. 3 (January 17, 2003): 1728–1734.

13. Ballinger, S.W., C. Patterson, C.N. Yan, R. Doan, D.L. Burow, C.G. Young, F.M. Yakes, et al. "Hydrogen peroxide- and peroxynitrite-induced mitochondrial DNA damage and dysfunction in vascular endothelial and smooth muscle cells." *Circulation Research* 86, no. 9 (May 12, 2000): 960–966.

14. Guo, C., L. Sun, X. Chen, and D. Zhang. "Oxidative stress, mito-chondrial damage and neurodegenerative diseases." *Neural Regeneration Research* 8, no. 21 (July 25, 2013): 2003–2014.

15. Pizzino, G., N. Irrera, M. Cucinotta, G. Pallio, F. Mannino, V. Arcoraci, F. Squadrito, D. Altavilla, and A. Bitto. "Oxidative stress: Harms and benefits for human health." *Oxidative Medicine and Cellular Longevity* 2017 (2017): 8416763.

16. Ristow and Schmeisser. "Mitohormesis."

17. Li, X., T. Yang, and Z. Sun. "Hormesis in health and chronic diseases." *Trends in Endocrinology & Metabolism* 30, no. 12 (December 2019): 944–958.

18. van Horssen, J., P. van Schaik, and M. Witte. "Inflammation and mitochondrial dysfunction: A vicious circle in neurodegenerative disorders?" *Neuroscience Letters* 710 (September 2019): 132931.

19. Suzuki, K., T. Tominaga, R.T. Ruhee, and S. Ma. "Characterization and modulation of systemic inflammatory response to exhaustive exercise in relation to oxidative stress." *Antioxidants* 9, no. 5 (May 8, 2020): 401.

20. Picard, M., B.S. McEwen, E.S. Epel, and C. Sandi. "An energetic view of stress: Focus on mitochondria." *Frontiers in Neuroendocrinology* 49 (April 2018): 72–85.

21. Brand, S., K. Ebner, T. Mikoteit, I. Lejri, M. Gerber, J. Beck, E. Holsboer-Trachsler, and A. Eckert. "Influence of regular physical activity on mitochondrial activity and symptoms of burnout—an interventional pilot study." *Journal of Clinical Medicine* 9, no. 3 (March 2, 2020): 667.

22. "Hardwired for laziness? Tests show the human brain must work hard to avoid sloth." Faculty of Medicine. University of British Columbia (September 18, 2018). https://www.med.ubc.ca/news/hardwired-for-laziness-tests-show-the-human-brain-must-work-hard-to-avoid-sloth.

23. Schwartz, M. "The benefits of fasting for a healthy gut." *Health*. (September 24, 2020). https://www.health.com/nutrition/how-to-fast-healthy-gut.

24. de Cabo, R., and M.P. Mattson. "Effects of intermittent fasting on health, aging, and disease." *New England Journal of Medicine* 381, no. 26 (December 16, 2019): 2541–2551.

25. Malinowski, B., K. Zalewska, A. Węsierska, M.M. Sokołowska, M. Socha, G. Liczner, K. Pawlak-Osińska, and M. Wiciński. "Intermittent fasting in cardiovascular disorders—an overview." *Nutrients* 11, no. 3 (March 20, 2019): 673.

26. Wang, X., Q. Yang, Q. Liao, M. Li, P. Zhang, H.O. Santos, H. Kord-Varkaneh, and M. Abshirini. "Effects of intermittent fasting diets on plasma concentrations of inflammatory biomarkers: A systematic review and meta-analysis of randomized controlled trials." *Nutrition* 2020, no. 79–80 (November–December 2020): 110974.

27. Halpern, B., and T.B. Mendes. "Intermittent fasting for obesity and related disorders: Unveiling myths, facts, and presumptions." *Archives of Endocrinology and Metabolism* 65 (January 18, 2021): 14–23.

28. Anton, S.D., K. Moehl, W.T. Donahoo, K. Marosi, S. Lee, A.G. Mainous, C. Leeuwenburgh, and M.P. Mattson. "Flipping the metabolic switch: Understanding and applying health benefits of fasting." *Obesity* (Silver Spring, MD) 26, no. 2 (February 2018): 254–268.

29. Anton et al. "Flipping the metabolic switch."

30. Orlich, M.J., J. Sabaté, A. Mashchak, U. Fresán, K. Jaceldo-Siegl, F. Miles, and G.E. Fraser. "Ultra-processed food intake and animal-based food intake and mortality in the Adventist Health Study-2." *American Journal of Clinical Nutrition* 115, no. 6 (June 1, 2022): 1589–1601.

31. Wilhelmi de Toledo, F., F. Grundler, A. Bergouignan, S. Drinda, and A. Michalsen. "Safety, health improvement and well-being during a 4 to 21-day fasting period in an observational study including 1422 subjects." *PLoS ONE* 14, no. 1 (January 2, 2019): e0209353.

32. Oksala, N.K.J., F.G. Ekmekçi, E. Özsoy, S. Kirankaya, T. Kokkola, G. Emecen, J. Lappalainen, K. Kaarniranta, and M. Atalay. "Natural thermal adaptation increases heat shock protein levels and decreases oxidative stress." *Redox Biology* no. 3 (October 24, 2014): 25–28.

33. Patrick, R.P., and T.L. Johnson. "Sauna use as a lifestyle practice to extend healthspan." *Experimental Gerontology* 154 (October 15, 2021): 111509.

34. Patrick and Johnson. "Sauna use as a lifestyle practice."

35. Hafen, P.S., C.N. Preece, J.R. Sorensen, C.R. Hancock, and R.D. Hyldahl. "Repeated exposure to heat stress induces mitochondrial adaptation in human skeletal muscle." *Journal of Applied Physiology* (Bethesda, MD: 1985) 125, no. 5 (November 1, 2018): 1447–1455.

36. Laukkanen, J.A., and T. Laukkanen. "Sauna bathing and systemic inflammation." *European Journal of Epidemiology* 33, no. 3 (March 2018): 351–353.

37. Sutkowy, P., A. Woźniak, T. Boraczyński, C. Mila-Kierzenkowska, and M. Boraczyński. "The effect of a single Finnish sauna bath after aerobic exercise on the oxidative status in healthy men." *Scandinavian Journal of Clinical Laboratory Investigation* 74, no. 2 (March 1, 2014): 89–94.

38. Jardine, D.S. "Heat illness and heat stroke." *Pediatrics in Review* 28, no. 7 (July 1, 2007): 249–258.

39. Hesketh, K., S.O. Shepherd, J.A. Strauss, D.A. Low, R.J. Cooper, A.J.M. Wagenmakers, and M. Cocks. "Passive heat therapy in sedentary humans increases skeletal muscle capillarization and eNOS content but not mitochondrial density or GLUT4 content." *American Journal of Physiology: Heart and Circulatory Physiology* 317 (May 10, 2019): H114–H123. https://journals.physiology.org/doi/pdf/10.1152/ajpheart.00816.2018.

40. Patrick and Johnson. "Sauna use as a lifestyle practice."

41. Markham, J. "Cold showers after using a sauna: Are they good for you?" SaunaVerse (October 8, 2021). https://saunaverse.com/cold-showers-after-using-a-sauna.

42. Phadtare, S., J. Alsina, and M. Inouye. "Cold-shock response and cold-shock proteins." *Current Opinion in Microbiology* 2, no. 2 (April 1, 1999): 175–180.

43. de Oliveira Ottone, V., F. de Castro Magalhães, F. de Paula, N.C.P. Avelar, P.F. Aguiar, P.F. da Matta Sampaio, and T.C. Duarte. "The effect of different water immersion temperatures on post-exercise

parasympathetic reactivation." *PLoS ONE* 9, no. 12 (December 1, 2014): e113730.

44. Knechtle, B., Z. Waśkiewicz, C.V. Sousa, L. Hill, and P.T Nikolaidis. "Cold water swimming—benefits and risks: A narrative review." *International Journal of Environmental Research and Public Health* 17, no. 23 (December 2020): 8984.

45. Shevchuk, N. "Adapted cold shower as a potential treatment for depression." *Medical Hypotheses* no. 70 (February 1, 2008): 995–1001.

46. Park, E.H., S.W. Choi, and Y.K. Yang. "Cold-water immersion promotes antioxidant enzyme activation in elite taekwondo athletes." *Applied Science* 2021 (March 23, 2021). https://doi.org/10.3390 /app11062855.

47. Lubkowska, A., B. Dołęgowska, Z. Szyguła, I. Bryczkowska, M. Stańczyk-Dunaj, D. Sałata, and M. Budkowska. "Winter-swimming as a building-up body resistance factor inducing adaptive changes in the oxidant/antioxidant status." *Scandinavian Journal of Clinical and Laboratory Investigation* 73, no. 4 (June 1, 2013): 315–325.

48. Allan, R., A.P. Sharples, G.L. Close, B. Drust, S.O. Shepherd, J. Dutton, J.P. Morten, and W. Gregson. "Postexercise cold water immersion modulates skeletal muscle PGC-1α mRNA expression in immersed and nonimmersed limbs: Evidence of systemic regulation." *Journal of Applied Physiology* (Bethesda, MD: 1985) 123, no. 2 (August 1, 2017): 451–459.

49. Joo, C.H., R. Allan, B. Drust, G.L. Close, T.S. Jeong, J.D. Bartlett, C. Mawhinney, J. Louhelainen, J.P. Morton, and W. Gregson. "Passive and post-exercise cold-water immersion augments PGC-1α and VEGF expression in human skeletal muscle." *European Journal of Applied Physiology* 116, no. 11–12 (December 2016): 2315–2326.

50. Ihsan, M., J.F. Markworth, G. Watson, H.C. Choo, A. Govus, T. Pham, A. Hickey, D. Cameron-Smith, and C.R. Abbiss. "Regular postexercise cooling enhances mitochondrial biogenesis through AMPK and p38 MAPK in human skeletal muscle." *American Journal of Physiology: Regulatory Integrative and Comparative Physiology* 309, no. 3 (August 2015): R286–R294.

51. Virtanen, K.A., M.E. Lidell, J. Orava, M. Heglind, R. Westergren, T. Niemi, M. Taittonen, et al. "Functional brown adipose tissue in

healthy adults." *New England Journal of Medicine* 360, no. 15 (April 9, 2009): 1518–1525.

52. Søberg, S., J. Löfgren, F.E. Philipsen, M. Jensen, A.E. Hansen, E. Ahrens, K.B. Nystrup, et al. "Altered brown fat thermoregulation and enhanced cold-induced thermogenesis in young, healthy, winter-swimming men." *Cell Reports: Medicine* 2, no. 10 (October 19, 2021): 100408.

53. "Cold exposure." FoundMyFitness. [Accessed July 28, 2022.] https://www.foundmyfitness.com/topics/cold-exposure-therapy.

54. Buijze, G.A., I.N. Sierevelt, B.C.J.M. van der Heijden, M.G. Dijkgraaf, and M.H.W Frings-Dresen. "The effect of cold showering on health and work: A randomized controlled trial." *PLoS ONE* 11, no. 9 (September 15, 2016): e0161749.

55. Allen, J.J. "Characteristics of users and reported effects of the Wim Hof method : A mixed-methods study." Student thesis. University of Twente (2018). [Accessed July 28, 2022.] http://essay.utwente.nl/76839.

56. Bleakley, C., S. McDonough, E. Gardner, G.D. Baxter, J.T. Hopkins, and G.W. Davison. "Cold-water immersion (cryotherapy) for preventing and treating muscle soreness after exercise." *Cochrane Database of Systematic Reviews* 2 (February 15, 2012): CD008262.

57. Park, Choi, and Yang. "Cold-water immersion."

58. Knechtle et al. "Cold water swimming."

59. Stanborough, R.J. "What to know about cold water therapy." *Healthline* (July 8, 2020). https://www.healthline.com/health/cold-water-therapy.

60. "Cold exposure." FoundMyFitness.

61. Hoffman, P.T. "How long does it take to get hypothermia in cold water?" Hofmann & Schweitzer law firm (June 2, 2022). https://www.hofmannlawfirm.com/faqs/how-long-does-it-take-to-get-hypothermia-in-cold-water.cfm.

62. Rew, K. "Afterdrop & the subtle art of warming up." The Outdoor Swimming Society. [Accessed July 28, 2022.] https://www.outdoorswimmingsociety.com/warming-up-after-drop.

63. Wimalawansa, S.J. "Vitamin D deficiency: Effects on oxidative stress, epigenetics, gene regulation, and aging." *Biology* (Basel, CH) 8, no. 2 (May 11, 2019): 30.

64. Hart, P.H., and S. Gorman. "Exposure to UV wavelengths in sunlight suppresses immunity. To what extent is UV-induced vitamin D3 the mediator responsible?" *Clinical Biochemical Reviews* 34, no. 1 (February 2013): 3–13.

65. Erem, A.S., and M.S. Razzaque. "Vitamin D-independent benefits of safe sunlight exposure." *Journal of Steroid Biochemistry and Molecular Biology* 213 (October 2021): 105957.

66. Holick, M.F. "Vitamin D deficiency in 2010: Health benefits of vitamin D and sunlight: A D-bate." *Nature Reviews: Endocrinology* 7, no. 2 (February 2011): 73–75.

67. National Institutes of Health researchers make a case: Office of Dietary Supplements. "Vitamin D: Fact sheet for health professionals." National Institutes of Health (June 2, 2022). https://ods.od.nih .gov/factsheets/VitaminD-HealthProfessional.

68. Wimalawansa. "Vitamin D deficiency."

69. Juzeniene, A., and J. Moan. "Beneficial effects of UV radiation other than via vitamin D production." *Dermato-endocrinology* 4, no. 2 (April 1, 2021): 109–117.

70. Sommer, A.P., P. Schemmer, A.E. Pavláth, H.D. Försterling, A.R. Mester, and M.A. Trelles. "Quantum biology in low level light therapy: Death of a dogma." *Annals of Translational Medicine* 8, no. 7 (April 2020): 440.

71. Sommer, A.P. "Mitochondrial solar sensitivity: Evolutionary and biomedical implications." *Annals of Translational Medicine* 8, no. 5 (March 2020): 161.

72. Sansone, R.A., and L.A. Sansone. "Sunshine, serotonin, and skin: A partial explanation for seasonal patterns in psychopathology?" *Innovations in Clinical Neuroscience* 10, no. 7–8 (July 2013): 20–24.

73. Hart and Gorman. "Exposure to UV wavelengths."

74. Autier, P., and J.F. Doré. "Ultraviolet radiation and cutaneous melanoma: A historical perspective." *Melanoma Research* 30, no. 2 (April 2020): 113–125.

75. "Vitamin D." Hot Topics. MS Society of Canada. [Accessed July 5, 2022.] https://mssociety.ca/hot-topics/vitamin-d.

76. Neale, R.E., S.R. Khan, R.M. Lucas, M. Waterhouse, D.C. Whiteman, and C.M. Olsen. "The effect of sunscreen on vitamin D: A review." *British Journal of Dermatology* 181, no. 5 (November 2019): 907–915.

77. McNeill, A.M., and E. Wesner. "Sun protection and vitamin D." The Skin Cancer Foundation (May 14, 2018). https://www.skincancer.org/blog/sun-protection-and-vitamin-d.

78. Adamson, A.S., and K. Shinkai. "Systemic absorption of sunscreen: Balancing benefits with unknown harms." *Journal of the American Medical Association* 323, no. 3 (January 21, 2020): 223–224.

79. *APA Dictionary of Psychology*. American Psychological Association. [Accessed July 14, 2022.] https://dictionary.apa.org.

80. Anderson, R., S.J. Hanrahan, and C.J. Mallett. "Investigating the optimal psychological state for peak performance in Australian elite athletes." *Journal of Applied Sport Psychology* 26, no. 3 (July 3, 2014): 318–333.

81. Cohen, R.A. "Yerkes–Dodson law." In *Encyclopedia of Clinical Neuropsychology*, ed. J.S. Kreutzer, J. DeLuca, and B. Caplan, 2737–2768 (New York: Springer, 2011).

82. May, K.E., and A.D. Elder. "Efficient, helpful, or distracting? A literature review of media multitasking in relation to academic performance." *International Journal of Educational Technology in Higher Education* 15, no. 1 (February 27, 2018): 13.

83. Adams, K. "We asked sports psychologists to analyze 5 Olympians' favourite pump-up songs." CBC Music (February 8, 2022). https://www.cbc.ca/music/we-asked-sports-psychologists-to-analyze-5-olympians-favourite-pump-up-songs-1.6353760.

84. Taylor, J. "How do you psych up when you get down in a competition?" Sports: Psych-up Techniques. *Psychology Today* (May 7, 2010). https://www.psychologytoday.com/us/blog/the-power-prime/201005/sports-psych-techniques.

85. "6 real mantras used by elite athletes." Fitness: Health. Built for Athletes (June 4, 2020). https://builtforathletes.com/blogs/news/6-real-mantras-used-by-elite-athletes.

86. Jiang, S., H. Liu, and C. Li. "Dietary regulation of oxidative stress in chronic metabolic diseases." *Foods* 10, no. 8 (August 11, 2021): 1854.

87. Pirouzeh, R., N. Heidarzadeh-Esfahani, M. Morvaridzadeh, A. Izadi, S. Yosaee, E. Potter, J. Heshmati, A.B. Pizarro, A. Omidi, and S. Heshmati. "Effect of DASH diet on oxidative stress parameters: A systematic review and meta-analysis of randomized clinical trials." *Diabetes and Metabolic Syndrome* 14, no. 6 (November–December 2020): 2131–2138.

88. Zeb, A. "Concept, mechanism, and applications of phenolic antioxidants in foods." *Journal of Food Biochemistry* 44, no. 9 (2020): e13394.

89. Tibullo, D., G. Li Volti, C. Giallongo, S. Grasso, D. Tomassoni, C.D. Anfuso, G. Lupo, F. Amenta, R. Avola, and V. Bramanti. "Biochemical and clinical relevance of alpha lipoic acid: Antioxidant and anti-inflammatory activity, molecular pathways and therapeutic potential." *Inflammation Research* 66, no. 11 (November 2017): 947–959.

90. Herbst, E.A.F., S. Paglialunga, C. Gerling, J. Whitfield, K. Mukai, A. Chabowski, G.J.F. Heigenhauser, L.L. Spriet, and G.P. Holloway. "Omega-3 supplementation alters mitochondrial membrane composition and respiration kinetics in human skeletal muscle." *Journal of Physiology* 592, pt. 6 (March 15, 2014): 1341–1352.

91. Xiao, B., Y. Li, Y. Lin, J. Lin, L. Zhang, D. Wu, J. Zeng, J. Li, J.W. Liu, and G. Li. "Eicosapentaenoic acid (EPA) exhibits antioxidant activity via mitochondrial modulation." *Food Chemistry* 373, pt. A (March 30, 2022): 131389.

92. Tan, B.L., M.E. Norhaizan, and W.P.P. Liew. "Nutrients and oxidative stress: Friend or foe?" *Oxidative Medicine and Cellular Longevity* 2018 (January 31, 2018): e9719584.

93. O'Sullivan, T.A., K. Hafekost, F. Mitrou, and D. Lawrence. "Food sources of saturated fat and the association with mortality: A meta-analysis." *American Journal of Public Health* 103, no. 9 (September 2013): e31–e42.

94. García-Closas, R., A. Berenguer, M.J. Tormo, M.J. Sánchez, J.R. Quirós, C. Navarro, R. Arnaud, et al. "Dietary sources of vitamin C, vitamin E and specific carotenoids in Spain." *British Journal of Nutrition* 91, no. 6 (June 2004): 1005–1011.

95. Olechnowicz, J., A. Tinkov, A. Skalny, and J. Suliburska. "Zinc status is associated with inflammation, oxidative stress, lipid, and glucose metabolism." *Journal of Physiological Sciences* 68, no. 1 (January 2018): 19–31.

96. Willcox, D.C., G. Scapagnini, and B.J. Willcox. "Healthy aging diets other than the Mediterranean: A focus on the Okinawan diet." *Mechanisms of Ageing and Development* 136–137 (March–April 2014): 148–162.

97. Zhang, Y.J., R.Y. Gan, S. Li, Y. Zhou, A.N. Li, D.P. Xu, and H.B. Li. "Antioxidant phytochemicals for the prevention and treatment of chronic diseases." *Molecules* 20, no. 12 (November 27, 2015): 21138–21156.

98. Silva, R.F.M., and L. Pogačnik. "Polyphenols from food and natural products: Neuroprotection and safety." *Antioxidants* (Basel, CH) 9, no. 1 (January 10, 2020): 61.

99. Pravst, I., K. Zmitek, and J. Zmitek. "Coenzyme Q10 contents in foods and fortification strategies." *Critical Reviews in Food Science and Nutrition* 50, no. 4 (April 2010): 269–280.

100. Hernández-Camacho, J.D., M. Bernier, G. López-Lluch, and P. Navas. "Coenzyme Q10 supplementation in aging and disease." *Frontiers in Physiology* 2018 (February 5, 2018): 9.

101. Hidalgo-Gutiérrez, A., P. González-García, M.E. Díaz-Casado, E. Barriocanal-Casado, S. López-Herrador, C.M. Quinzii, and L.C. López. "Metabolic targets of coenzyme Q10 in mitochondria." *Antioxidants* (Basel, CH) 10, no. 4 (March 26, 2021): 520.

102. Jonscher, K.R., and R.B. Rucker. "Chapter 13. Pyrroloquinoline quinone: Its profile, effects on the liver and implications for health and disease prevention." *Dietary Interventions in Liver Disease* 2019 (February 8, 2019): 157–173. https://www.sciencedirect.com/science/article/pii/B9780128144664000136.

103. Harris, C.B., W. Chowanadisai, D.O. Mishchuk, M.A. Satre, C.M. Slupsky, and R.B. Rucker. "Dietary pyrroloquinoline quinone (PQQ) alters indicators of inflammation and mitochondrial-related metabolism in human subjects." *Journal of Nutritional Biochemistry* 24, no. 12 (December 2013): 2076–2084.

104. Jones, D.P., R.J. Coates, E.W. Flagg, J.W. Eley, G. Block, R.S. Greenberg, E.W. Gunter, and B. Jackson. "Glutathione in foods listed in the National Cancer Institute's Health Habits and History Food Frequency Questionnaire." *Nutrition and Cancer* 17, no. 1 (1992): 57–75.

105. Wood, A.M., J.J. Froh, and A.W. Geraghty. "Gratitude and well-being: A review and theoretical integration." *Clinical Psychology Review* 30, no. 7 (November 2010): 890–905.

106. "Gratitude is good medicine." UC Davis Health (November 25, 2015). https://health.ucdavis.edu/medicalcenter/features/2015-2016/11/20151125_gratitude.html.

107. Simon-Thomas, E.R., and K.M. Newman. "How happy are people at work?" *Greater Good Magazine* (July 10, 2019). https://greatergood.berkeley.edu/article/item/how_happy_are_people_at_work.

108. Picard, M., A.A. Prather, E. Puterman, A. Cuillerier, M. Coccia, K. Aschbacher, Y. Burelle, and E.S. Epel. "A mitochondrial health index sensitive to mood and caregiving stress." *Biological Psychiatry* 84, no. 1 (July 1, 2018): 9–17.

109. Selva, J. "Gratitude meditation: A simple but powerful happiness intervention." Gratitude. PositivePsychology.com (April 21, 2017). https://positivepsychology.com/gratitude-meditation-happiness.

110. Altruism. *Psychology Today*. [Accessed July 26, 2022.] https://www.psychologytoday.com/ca/basics/altruism.

111. Savulescu, J., and W. Sinnott-Armstrong. "Five ways to become a really effective altruist." *The Conversation* (February 8, 2016). http://theconversation.com/five-ways-to-become-a-really-effective-altruist-53684.

112. Barragan, R.C., R. Brooks, and A.N. Meltzoff. "Altruistic food sharing behavior by human infants after a hunger manipulation." *Scientific Reports* 10, no. 1 (February 4, 2020): 1785.

113. Altruism. *Psychology Today*.

114. Filkowski, M.M., R.M. Cochran, and B.W. Haas. "Altruistic behavior: Mapping responses in the brain." *Neuroscience and Neuroeconomics* 5 (2016): 65–75.

115. Picard, M., and C. Sandi. "The social nature of mitochondria: Implications for human health." *Neuroscience and Biobehavioral Reviews* 120 (January 2021): 595–610.

116. Theoharides, T.C. "On the gut microbiome-brain axis and altruism." *Clinical Therapeutics* 37, no. 5 (May 1, 2015): 937–940.

117. Picard and Sandi. "The social nature of mitochondria."

118. Post, S.G. (ed.) *Altruism and Health: Perspectives from Empirical Research* (New York: Oxford University Press, 2007).

119. Picard and Sandi. "The social nature of mitochondria."

120. Post. *Altruism and Health*.

121. Post, S.G. "Altruism, happiness, and health: It's good to be good." *International Journal of Behavioral Medicine* 12, no. 2 (2005): 66–77.

122. Hu, T.Y., J. Li, H. Jia, and X. Xie. "Helping others, warming yourself: Altruistic behaviors increase warmth feelings of the ambient environment." *Frontiers in Psychology* 7 (September 5, 2016): 1349.

123. Wang, Y., J. Ge, H. Zhang, H. Wang, and X. Xie. "Altruistic behaviors relieve physical pain." *Proceedings of the National Academy of Sciences of the United States of America* 117, no. 2 (January 14, 2020): 950–958.

124. Post, S.G. "Six ways to boost your 'habits of helping.'" *Greater Good Magazine* (March 15, 2011). https://greatergood.berkeley.edu/article/item/six_ways_to_become_more_altruistic.

125. "Eliciting altruism: How to overcome barriers to kindness in yourself and others." Greater Good in Action. [Accessed July 27, 2022.] https://ggia.berkeley.edu/index.php/practice/eliciting_altruism.

Chapter 4: Thrive

1. Chan, J., and S. Clarke. *2021 Workplace Burnout Study*. Infinite Potential. [Accessed October 6, 2022.] https://img1.wsimg.com/blobby/go/6c37d4f0-7b8a-4dd3-afb8-0a1b504af624/2021%20Workplace%20Burnout%20Study-%20Final.pdf.

2. Brown, D.J., R. Arnold, D. Fletcher, and M. Standage. "Human thriving: A conceptual debate and literature review." *European Psychology* 22, no. 3 (July 2017): 167–179.

3. Su, R., L. Tay, and E. Diener. "The development and validation of the Comprehensive Inventory of Thriving (CIT) and the Brief Inventory of Thriving (BIT)." *Applied Psychology: Health and Well-Being* 6, no. 3 (November 2014): 251–279.

4. Feeney, B.C., and N.L. Collins. "A new look at social support: A theoretical perspective on thriving through relationships." *Personality and Social Psychology Review* 19, no. 2 (May 2015): 113–147.

5. Winkel, A.F., A.W. Honart, A. Robinson, A.A. Jones, and A. Squires. "Thriving in scrubs: A qualitative study of resident resilience." *Reproductive Health* 15, no. 1 (December 2018): 53.

6. Stoffle, C.J., and C. Cuillier. "From surviving to thriving." *Journal of Library Administration* 51, no. 1 (December 30, 2010): 130–155.

7. Park, C.L., L.H. Cohen, and R.L. Murch. "Assessment and prediction of stress-related growth." *Journal of Personality* 64, no. 1 (March 1996): 71–105.

8. Niemiec, R.M. "Six functions of character strengths for thriving at times of adversity and opportunity: A theoretical perspective." *Applied Research in Quality of Life* 15, no. 2 (April 1, 2020): 551–572.

9. Ding, W.X., and X.M. Yin. "Mitophagy: Mechanisms, pathophysiological roles, and analysis." *Biological Chemistry* 393, no. 7 (July 2012): 547–564.

10. Murali Mahadevan, H., A. Hashemiaghdam, G. Ashrafi, and A.B. Harbauer. "Mitochondria in neuronal health: From energy metabolism to Parkinson's disease." *Advanced Biology* (Weinh) 5, no. 9 (September 2021): e2100663.

11. Schapira, A.H. "Mitochondrial involvement in Parkinson's disease, Huntington's disease, hereditary spastic paraplegia and Friedreich's ataxia." *Biochimica et Biophysica Acta* 1410, no. 2 (February 9, 1999): 159–170.

12. Murphy, M.P., and R.C. Hartley. "Mitochondria as a therapeutic target for common pathologies." *Nature Reviews: Drug Discovery* 17, no. 12 (December 2018): 865–886.

13. Briston, T., and A.R. Hicks. "Mitochondrial dysfunction and neurodegenerative proteinopathies: Mechanisms and prospects for therapeutic intervention." *Biochemical Society Transactions* 46, no. 4 (August 20, 2018): 829–842.

14. Lin, M.T., and M.F. Beal. "Mitochondrial dysfunction and oxidative stress in neurodegenerative diseases." *Nature* 443, no. 7113 (October 19, 2006): 787–795.

15. Andreux, P.A., R.H. Houtkooper, and J. Auwerx. "Pharmacological approaches to restore mitochondrial function." *Nature Reviews: Drug Discovery* 12, no. 6 (June 2013): 465–483.

16. Elfawy, H.A., and B. Das. "Crosstalk between mitochondrial dysfunction, oxidative stress, and age related neurodegenerative disease: Etiologies and therapeutic strategies." *Life Sciences* 218 (February 1, 2019): 165–184.

17. Rocha, E.M., B. De Miranda, and L.H. Sanders. "Alpha-synuclein: Pathology, mitochondrial dysfunction and neuroinflammation in Parkinson's disease." *Neurobiology of Disease* 109, pt. B (January 2018): 249–257.

18. Macdonald, R., K. Barnes, C. Hastings, and H. Mortiboys. "Mitochondrial abnormalities in Parkinson's disease and Alzheimer's disease: Can mitochondria be targeted therapeutically?" *Biochemical Society Transactions* 46, no. 4 (August 20, 2018): 891–909.

19. Lekkas, D., J.A. Gyorda, G.D. Price, Z. Wortzman, and N.C. Jacobson. "Using the COVID-19 pandemic to assess the influence of news affect on online mental health-related search behavior across the United States: Integrated sentiment analysis and the circumplex model of affect." *Journal of Medical Internet Research* 24, no. 1 (January 27, 2022): e32731.

20. Grant, A. "There's a name for the blah you're feeling: It's called languishing." *New York Times* (April 19, 2021). https://www.nytimes.com/2021/04/19/well/mind/covid-mental-health-languishing.html.

21. Keyes, C.L. "The mental health continuum: From languishing to flourishing in life." *Journal of Health and Social Behavior* 43, no. 2 (June 2002): 207–222.

22. Keyes, C.L., S.S. Dhingra, and E.J. Simoes. "Change in level of positive mental health as a predictor of future risk of mental illness." *American Journal of Public Health* 100, no. 12 (December 2010): 2366–2371.

23. Bassi, M., L. Negri, A. Delle Fave, and R. Accardi. "The relationship between post-traumatic stress and positive mental health symptoms among health workers during COVID-19 pandemic in Lombardy, Italy." *Journal of Affected Disorders* 280, pt. B (February 1, 2021): 1–6.

24. Knoesen, R., and L. Naudé. "Experiences of flourishing and languishing during the first year at university." *Journal of Mental Health* (Abingdon, UK) 27, no. 3 (June 2018): 269–278.

25. Gloster, A.T., D. Lamnisos, J. Lubenko, G. Presti, V. Squatrito, M. Constantinou, C. Nicolaou, et al. "Impact of COVID-19 pandemic on mental health: An international study." *PloS One* 15, no. 12 (December 31, 2020): e0244809.

26. Iasiello, M., J. van Agteren, C.L.M. Keyes, and E.M. Cochrane. "Positive mental health as a predictor of recovery from mental illness." *Journal of Affective Disorders* 251 (May 15, 2019): 227–230.

27. Willen, S.S., A.F. Williamson, C.C. Walsh, M. Hyman, and W. Tootle. "Rethinking flourishing: Critical insights and qualitative perspectives from the U.S. Midwest." *SSM Mental Health* 2 (December 2022): 100057.

28. Fredrickson, B.L., and M.F. Losada. "Positive affect and the complex dynamics of human flourishing." *American Psychology* 60, no. 7 (October 2005): 678–686.

29. Keyes. "The mental health continuum."

30. "Mental Health." Health Topics. World Health Organization. [Accessed June 15, 2022.] https://www.who.int/health-topics/mental-health#tab=tab_1.

31. Eraslan-Capan, B. "Social connectedness and flourishing: The mediating role of hopelessness." *Universal Journal of Educational Research* 4, no. 5 (May 2016): 933–940.

32. Ho, H.C.Y., and Y.C. Chan. "Flourishing in the workplace: A one-year prospective study on the effects of perceived organizational support and psychological capital." *International Journal of Environmental Research and Public Health* 19, no. 2 (January 14, 2022): 922.

33. In an article for the *New York Times*, Gretchen Reynolds makes a case: Reynolds, G. "How exercise may help us flourish." *New York Times* (May 12, 2021). https://www.nytimes.com/2021/05/12/well /move/exercise-mental-health-flourishing.html.

34. Yemiscigil, A., and I. Vlaev. "The bidirectional relationship between sense of purpose in life and physical activity: A longitudinal study." *Journal of Behavioral Medicine* 44, no. 5 (October 2021): 715–725.

35. Leibow, M.S., J.W. Lee, and K.R. Morton. "Exercise, flourishing, and the positivity ratio in Seventh-Day Adventists: A prospective study." *American Journal of Health Promotion* 35, no. 1 (January 2021): 48–56.

36. Bzdok, D., and R.I.M. Dunbar. "The neurobiology of social distance." *Trends in Cognitive Sciences* 24, no. 9 (September 2020): 717–733.

37. Holt-Lunstad, J. "Loneliness and social isolation as risk factors: The power of social connection in prevention." *American Journal of Lifestyle Medicine* 15, no. 5 (May 6, 2021): 567–573.

38. Flannery, M. "Self-determination theory: Intrinsic motivation and behavioral change." *Oncology Nursing Forum* 44, no. 2 (March 1, 2017): 155–156.

39. Cruwys, T., G.A. Dingle, C. Haslam, S.A. Haslam, J. Jetten, and T.A. Morton. "Social group memberships protect against future depression, alleviate depression symptoms and prevent depression relapse." *Social Science and Medicine* (1982) 98 (December 2013): 179–186.

40. Jones, J.M., W.H. Williams, J. Jetten, S.A. Haslam, A. Harris, and H. Gleibs. "The role of psychological symptoms and social group memberships in the development of post-traumatic stress after traumatic injury." *British Journal of Health Psychology* 17, no. 4 (November 2012): 798–811.

41. Shaya, F.T., V.V. Chirikov, D. Howard, C. Foster, J. Costas, S. Snitker, J. Frimpter, and K. Kucharski. "Effect of social networks intervention in type 2 diabetes: A partial randomised study." *Journal of Epidemiology and Community Health* 68, no. 4 (April 2014): 326–332.

42. Welin, L., B. Larsson, K. Svärdsudd, B. Tibblin, and G. Tibblin. "Social network and activities in relation to mortality from cardiovascular diseases, cancer and other causes: A 12 year follow up of the study of men born in 1913 and 1923." *Journal of Epidemiology and Community Health* 46, no. 2 (April 1992): 127–132.

43. Spiegel, D., J.R. Bloom, H.C. Kraemer, and E. Gottheil. "Effect of psychosocial treatment on survival of patients with metastatic breast cancer." Clinical Trial. *Lancet* (London) 2, no. 8668 (October 14, 1989): 888–891.

44. Floud, S., A. Balkwill, D. Canoy, F.L. Wright, G.K. Reeves, J. Green, V. Beral, B.J. Cairns, and the Million Women Study Collaborators. "Marital status and ischemic heart disease incidence and mortality in women: A large prospective study." *BMC Medicine* 12 (March 12, 2014): 42.

45. Holt-Lunstad, J., T.B. Smith, and J.B. Layton. "Social relationships and mortality risk: A meta-analytic review." *PloS Medicine* 7, no. 7 (2010): e1000316.

46. Pressman, S.D., S. Cohen, G.E. Miller, A. Barkin, B.S. Rabin, and J.J. Treanor. "Loneliness, social network size, and immune response to influenza vaccination in college freshmen." *Health Psychology* 24, no. 3 (May 2005): 297–306.

47. Martino, J., J. Pegg, and E.P. Frates. "The connection prescription: Using the power of social interactions and the deep desire for connectedness to empower health and wellness." *American Journal of Lifestyle Medicine* 11, no. 6 (October 7, 2015): 466–475.

48. Luenendonk, M. "Why your inner circle should stay small, and how to shrink it." Cleverism (November 26, 2020). https://www.cleverism .com/why-your-inner-circle-should-stay-small-and-how-to-shrink-it.

49. Holt-Lunstad, J. "Why social relationships are important for physical health: A systems approach to understanding and modifying risk and protection." *Annual Review of Psychology* 69 (January 4, 2018): 437–458.

50. Lin, C. " How young is too young for social media? Behavioral scientists are closer to an answer." Fast Company (October 29, 2021). https://www.fastcompany.com/90691317/kids-social-media-research-behavior.

51. Small, G.W., J. Lee, A. Kaufman, J. Jalil, P. Siddarth, H. Gaddipati, T.D. Moody, and S.Y. Bookheimer. "Brain health consequences of digital technology use." *Dialogues in Clinical Neuroscience* 22, no. 2 (June 2020): 179–187.

52. Brand, M. "Can internet use become addictive?" *Science* 376, no. 6595 (May 20, 2022): 798–799.

53. Firth, J., J. Torous, B. Stubbs, J.A. Firth, G.Z. Steiner, L. Smith, M. Alvarez-Jimenez, et al. "The 'online brain': How the internet may be changing our cognition." *World Psychiatry* 18, no. 2 (June 2019): 119–129.

54. Carter, B., P. Rees, L. Hale, D. Bhattacharjee, and M.S. Paradkar. "Association between portable screen-based media device access or use and sleep outcomes: A systematic review and meta-analysis." *JAMA Pediatrics* 170, no. 12 (December 1, 2016): 1202–1208.

55. Dong, G., and M.N. Potenza. "Behavioural and brain responses related to internet search and memory." *European Journal of Neuroscience* 42, no. 8 (October 2015): 2546–2554.

56. Duhigg, C. "The power of habit." [Accessed October 6, 2022.] https://charlesduhigg.com/the-power-of-habit.

57. Carter, B., P. Rees, L. Hale, D. Bhattacharjee, and M. Paradkar M. "A meta-analysis of the effect of media devices on sleep outcomes." *JAMA Pediatrics* 170, no. 12 (December 1, 2016): 1202–1208.

58. Dfarhud, D., M. Malmir, and M. Khanahmadi. "Happiness & health: The biological factors—systematic review article." *Iranian Journal of Public Health* 43, no. 11 (November 2014): 1468–1477.

59. Panagi, L., L. Poole, R.A. Hackett, and A. Steptoe. "Happiness and inflammatory responses to acute stress in people with type 2 diabetes." *Annals of Behavioral Medicine* 53, no. 4 (March 20, 2019): 309–320.

60. Salas-Vallina, A., M. Pozo-Hidalgo, and P.R. Gil-Monte. "Are happy workers more productive? The mediating role of service-skill use." *Frontiers in Psychology* 11 (March 27, 2020): 456.

61. Picard, M., A.A. Prather, E. Puterman, A. Cuillerier, M. Coccia, K. Aschbacher, Y. Burelle, and E.S. Epel. "A mitochondrial health index sensitive to mood and caregiving stress." *Biological Psychiatry* 84, no. 1 (July 1, 2018): 9–17.

62. Lyubomirsky, S., K.M. Sheldon, and D. Schkade. "Pursuing happiness: The architecture of sustainable change." *Review of General Psychology* 9, no. 2 (2005): 111–131. http://sonjalyubomirsky.com/wp-content/themes/sonjalyubomirsky/papers/LSS2005.pdf.

63. Gordon, N.S., S. Burke, H. Akil, S.J. Watson, and J. Panksepp. "Socially-induced brain 'fertilization': Play promotes brain derived neurotrophic factor transcription in the amygdala and dorsolateral frontal cortex in juvenile rats." *Neuroscience Letters* 341, no. 1 (April 24, 2003): 17–20.

64. Wood, A.M., J.J. Froh, and A.W.A. Geraghty. "Gratitude and well-being: A review and theoretical integration." *Clinical Psychology Review* 30, no. 7 (November 2010): 890–905.

65. Akimbekov, N.S., and M.S. Razzaque. "Laughter therapy: A humor-induced hormonal intervention to reduce stress and anxiety." *Current Research in Physiology* 4 (April 30, 2021): 135–138.

66. Gaines, J. "The philosophy of ikigai: 3 examples about finding purpose." Meaning & Values. Positive Phychology.com (November 17, 2020). https://positivepsychology.com/ikigai.

67. Mathews, G. "The stuff of dreams, fading: Ikigai and 'the Japanese self.'" *Ethos* 24, no. 4 (December 1996): 718–747.

68. Kotera, Y., G. Kaluzeviciute, G. Garip, K. McEwan, and K. Chamberlain. "Health benefits of ikigai: A review of literature." In *Ikigai: Towards a Psychological Understanding of a Life Worth Living*, ed. Y. Kotera and D. Fido, 1–13 (Toronto: Concurrent Disorders Society Press, 2021). https://repository.derby.ac.uk/item/92qzv/health-benefits-of-ikigai-a-review-of-literature.

69. Shirai, K., H. Iso, H. Fukuda, Y. Toyoda, T. Takatorige, and K. Tatara. "Factors associated with 'ikigai' among members of a public temporary employment agency for seniors (Silver Human Resources Centre) in Japan; gender differences." *Health and Quality of Life Outcomes* 4 (February 27, 2006): 12.

70. Kotera et al. "Health benefits of ikigai."

71. Kotera et al. "Health benefits of ikigai."

72. Wilkes, J., G. Garip, Y. Kotera, and D. Fido. "Can ikigai predict anxiety, depression, and well-being?" *International Journal of Mental Health Addiction* (March 1, 2022). https://doi.org/10.1007/s11469-022-00764-7.

73. Tanno, K., K. Sakata, M. Ohsawa, T. Onoda, K. Itai, Y. Yaegashi, A. Tamakoshi, and JACC Study Group. "Associations of ikigai as a pos-

itive psychological factor with all-cause mortality and cause-specific mortality among middle-aged and elderly Japanese people: Findings from the Japan Collaborative Cohort Study." *Journal of Psychosomatic Research* 67, no. 1 (July 2009): 67–75.

74. Mori, K., Y. Kaiho, Y. Tomata, M. Narita, F. Tanji, K. Sugiyama, Y. Sugawara, and I. Tsuji. "Sense of life worth living (ikigai) and incident functional disability in elderly Japanese: The Tsurugaya Project." *Journal of Psychosomatic Research* 95 (April 2017): 62–67. Erratum in *Journal of Psychosomatic Research* 96 (May 2017): 106.

75. Nakanishi, N., K. Tatara, F. Shinsho, T. Takatorige, S. Murakami, and H. Fukuda. "Prevalence of intellectual dysfunctioning and its correlates in a community-residing elderly population." *Scandinavian Journal of Social Medicine* 26, no. 3 (September 1998): 198–203.

76. Ishida, R., and M. Okada. "Effects of a firm purpose in life on anxiety and sympathetic nervous activity caused by emotional stress: Assessment by psycho-physiological method." *Stress and Health* 22, no. 4 (2006): 275–281.

77. Ishida, R. "Enormous earthquake in Japan: Coping with stress using purpose-in-life/ikigai. *Psychology* 2, no. 8 (November 4, 2011): 773–776.

78. Mogi, K. *The Little Book of Ikigai: The Secret Japanese Way to Live a Happy and Long Life* (London: Quercus Publishing, 2017).

79. Schippers, M.C., and N. Ziegler. "Life crafting as a way to find purpose and meaning in life." *Frontiers in Psychology* (December 13, 2019). https://www.frontiersin.org/articles/10.3389/fpsyg.2019.02778.

80. Fukuzawa, A., K. Katagiri, K. Harada, K. Masumoto, M. Chogahara, N. Kondo, and S. Okada. "A longitudinal study of the moderating effects of social capital on the relationships between changes in human capital and ikigai among Japanese older adults." *Asian Journal of Social Psychology* 22, no. 2 (2019): 172–182.

81. Lam, H.K.N., H. Middleton, and S.M. Phillips. "The effect of self-selected music on endurance running capacity and performance in a mentally fatigued state." *Journal of Human Sport and Exercise* 17, no. 4 (February 2021). https://doi.org/10.14198/jhse.2022.174.16.

82. Centala, J., C. Pogorel, S.W. Pummill, and M.H. Malek. "Listening to fast-tempo music delays the onset of neuromuscular fatigue." *Journal of Strength and Conditioning Research* 34, no. 3 (March 2020):

617–622.

83. Chanda, M.L., and D.J. Levitin. "The neurochemistry of music." *Trends in Cognitive Sciences* 17, no. 4 (April 2013): 179–193.

84. Patel, D. "These 6 types of music are known to dramatically improve productivity." Entrepreneur (January 9, 2019): https://www.entrepreneur.com/article/325492.

85. Habibi, A., A. Damasio, B. Ilari, M. Elliott Sachs, and H. Damasio. "Music training and child development: A review of recent findings from a longitudinal study." *Annals of the New York Academy of Sciences* 1423, no. 1 (March 6, 2018): 73–81.

86. Dukić, H. "Music, brain plasticity and the resilience: The pillars of new receptive therapy." *Psychiatria Danubina* 30, supp. 3 (April 2018): 141–147.

87. Feng, Q., L. Wang, Y. Chen, J. Teng, M. Li, Z. Cai, X. Nui, et al. "Effects of different music on HEK293T cell growth and mitochondrial functions." *EXPLORE* (January 10, 2022). https://www.sciencedirect.com/science/article/pii/S1550830722000027.

88. Chick, G., C. Yarnal, and A. Purrington. "Play and mate preference: Testing the signal theory of adult playfulness." *American Journal of Play* 4, no. 4 (2012): 407–440.

89. Wallace, J. "Why it's good for grown-ups to go play." Health and Science. *Washington Post* (May 20, 2017). https://www.washington-post.com/national/health-science/why-its-good-for-grown-ups-to-go-play/2017/05/19/99810292-fd1f-11e6-8ebe-6e0dbe4f2bca_story.html.

90. Magnuson, C.D., and L.A. Barnett. "The playful advantage: How playfulness enhances coping with stress." *Leisure Sciences* 35, no. 2 (2013): 129–144.

91. Neale, D. "A golden age of play for adults." British Psychological Society (March 25, 2020). https://www.bps.org.uk/psychologist/golden-age-play-adults.

92. Edwards, D. "Play and the feel good hormones." Primal Play (June 23, 2022). https://www.primalplay.com/blog/play-and-the-feel-good

-hormones.

93.   Guitard, P., F. Ferland, and É. Dutil. "Toward a better understanding of playfulness in adults." *OTJR: Occupation, Participation and Health* 25, no. 1 (January 1, 2005): 9–22.

94.   Fourie, L., C. Els, and L.T. De Beer. "A play-at-work intervention: What are the benefits?" *South African Journal of Economic Management Science* 23, no. 1 (January 2020): 1–11.

95.   Dresler, E., and P. Perera. "'Doing mindful colouring': Just a leisure activity or something more?" *Leisure Studies* 38, no. 6 (2019): 862–874.

96.   Fitzpatrick, K. "Why adult coloring books are good for you." CNN (August 1, 2017). https://www.cnn.com/2016/01/06/health/adult -coloring-books-popularity-mental-health/index.html.

97.   Moran, B. "Amazing benefits of puzzles for adults." Madd Capp Games (2020). [Accessed October 6, 2022.] https://maddcappgames .com/blogs/news/usa-today-on-the-benefits-of-puzzles-for-adults.

98.   "The cat's out of the bag: Animals play a big role in boosting our mental health." Canada Protection Plan (May 1, 2019). https://www .cpp.ca/blog/the-cats-out-of-the-bag-animals-play-a-big-role -in-boosting-our-mental-health.

99.   Manferdelli, G., A. La Torre, and R. Codella. "Outdoor physical activity bears multiple benefits to health and society." *Journal of Sports Medicine and Physical Fitness* 59, no. 5 (May 2019): 868–879.

100.   Gladwell, V.F., D.K. Brown, C. Wood, G.R. Sandercock, and J.L. Barton. "The great outdoors: How a green exercise environment can benefit all." *Extreme Physiological Medicine* 2, no. 1 (January 3, 2013): 3.

101.   Privette, G. "Chapter 14: Defining moments of self-actualization: Peak performance and peak experience." In *The Handbook of Humanistic Psychology: Leading Edges in Theory, Research, and Practice*, ed. K.J. Schneider, J.F.T. Bugental, and J.F. Pierson, 160–181 (New York: SAGE Publications, 2001). https://dx.doi.org/10.4135/9781412976268 .n14.

102.   Maslow, A. *Toward a Psychology of Being* (New York: Wiley, 1998).

INDEX